Review of Organic Functional Groups

Introduction to Medicinal Organic Chemistry

Fifth Edition

Thomas L. Lemke, Ph.D.
Professor Emeritus
College of Pharmacy
University of Houston
Houston, Texas

CASE AUTHORS:

Victoria F. Roche, Ph.D.
Senior Associate Dean
School of Pharmacy and Health
Professions
Creighton University
Omaha, Nebraska

S. William Zito, Ph.D.
Professor of Pharmaceutical Sciences
College of Pharmacy and Allied
Health Professions
St. John's University
Jamaica, New York

Wolters Kluwer | Lippincott Williams & Wilkins
Health
Philadelphia · Baltimore · New York · London
Buenos Aires · Hong Kong · Sydney · Tokyo

Senior Acquisitions Editor: David Troy
Managing Editor: Meredith Brittain
Product Managers: Meredith Brittain/Paula Williams
Marketing Manager: Allison Powell
Designer: Holly McLaughlin
Compositor: MPS Limited, A Macmillan Company

Fifth Edition

351 West Camden Street
Baltimore, MD 21201

Two Commerce Square
2001 Market Street
Philadelphia, PA 19106

Printed in theUnited States of America

9 8 7 6

Library of Congress Cataloging-in-Publication Data

Lemke, Thomas L.
Review of organic functional groups: introduction to medicinal organic chemistry/
Thomas L. Lemke.—5th ed.
    p. ; cm.
    Includes bibliographical references and index.
    ISBN 978-1-60831-016-6 (alk. paper)
    1. Pharmaceutical chemistry. I. Title.
    RS403.L397 2012
    615'.19—dc22

                                                2010023763

DISCLAIMER
Care has been taken to confirm the accuracy of the information present and to describe generally accepted practices. However, the authors, editors, and publisher are not responsible for errors or omissions or for any consequences from application of the information in this book and make no war-ranty, expressed or implied, with respect to the currency, completeness, or accuracy of the contents of the publication. Application of this information in a particular situation remains the professional responsibility of the practitioner; the clinical treatments described and recommended may not be considered absolute and universal recommendations.

The authors, editors, and publisher have exerted every effort to ensure that drug selection and dosage set forth in this text are in accordance with the current recommendations and practice at the time of publication. However, in view of ongoing research, changes in government regulations, and the constant flow of information relating to drug therapy and drug reactions, the reader is urged to check the package insert for each drug for any change in indications and dosage and for added warnings and precautions. This is particularly important when the recommended agent is a new or infrequently employed drug.

Some drugs and medical devices presented in this publication have Food and Drug Administration (FDA) clearance for limited use in restricted research settings. It is the responsibility of the health care provider to ascertain the FDA status of each drug or device planned for use in their clinical practice.

To purchase additional copies of this book, call our customer service department at **(800) 638-3030** or fax orders to **(301) 223-2320**. International customers should call **(301) 223-2300**.

Visit Lippincott Williams & Wilkins on the Internet: http://www.lww.com. Lippincott Williams & Wilkins customer service representatives are available from 8:30 am to 6:00 pm, EST.

Preface

This book has been prepared with the intent that it may be used as a self-paced review of organic functional groups. If the material covered in this book were to be presented in a conventional classroom setting, it would require 14 to 16 formal lecture hours. With this in mind, you should not attempt to cover all of the material in one sitting. A slow, leisurely pace will greatly increase your comprehension and decrease the number of return visits to the material. You should stop to review any section that you do not completely understand. You should also use the problem sets and detailed answers on the enclosed CD-ROM to enhance your understanding of the organic functional groups (Chapters 2–17). See the "Additional Resources" section, below, for more information.

OBJECTIVES

The book is designed as a review of the organic functional groups common to organic medicinal agents. It is the objective of this book to review the general topics of nomenclature, physical properties (with specific emphasis placed on water and lipid solubility), chemical properties (the stability or lack of stability of a functional group to normal environmental conditions, referred to as in vitro stability), and metabolism (the stability or lack of stability of a functional group in the body, referred to as in vivo stability). There will be no attempt to cover synthesis, nor will great emphasis be placed on chemical reactions except when they related to the physical or chemical stability and mechanistic action of drugs. This review is meant to provide background material for the formal pharmacy courses in medicinal chemistry. The objectives are presented in the following manner to aid in focusing attention on the expected learning outcomes.

- *Nomenclature*
  1. Common
  2. Official (IUPAC)°
  3. Generic (name of the functional group)
- *Physical-Chemical Properties*
  1. Physical properties—related to water and lipid solubility
  2. Chemical properties in vitro—stability or reactivity of functional groups "on the shelf"

°While IUPAC nomenclature will be presented for individual functional groups, it is normally not expected that a student will be able to draw a structure based upon IUPAC nomenclature of polyfunctional molecules (most drugs are polyfunctional), nor will the student be expected to write an IUPAC name based upon the chemical structure. The student is expected to identify the individual functional groups within a drug molecule using the common or generic name of the functional group.

- *Metabolism*
  Chemical properties in vivo—stability or reactivity of functional groups "in the body"

Upon successful completion of the book, the following general objectives will have been attained:

- The student will be able to draw a chemical structure of simple organic molecules given a common or official chemical name. With more complex polyfunctional molecules, the student will be able to identify functional groups (generic name) given the chemical structure.
- The student will be able to predict the solubility of a chemical in
  1. aqueous acid
  2. water
  3. aqueous base
- The student will be able to predict and show, with chemical structures, the chemical instabilities of each organic functional group under conditions appropriate to a substance "setting on the shelf," by which is meant conditions such as air, light, aqueous acid or base, and heat.
- The student will be able to predict and show, with chemical structures, the metabolism of each organic functional group.

A more detailed list of learning objectives can be found in Appendix D.

NEW TO THIS EDITION

The following features have been added to the fifth edition to enhance student understanding:

- **Case studies.** In Chapters 5 through 18, two cases per chapter will help prepare students in applying the material found in the book to clinical situations. Answers to the cases can be found on the CD packaged with this book.
- **Key terms** and a **glossary.** Important terms appear in boldface at their first appearance in the book and are defined in the glossary for handy reference.
- **Appendix D, Learning Objectives.** This appendix explains the knowledge and skills the student will have mastered after reading the book and doing the CD exercises.

RECOMMENDED PREPARATION

In order to maximize learning and to provide perspective in the study of the book, it would be helpful to read certain background material. It is highly recommended that a textbook on general organic chemistry be reviewed and consulted as a reference book while using this book. Pay special attention to the sections on nomenclature and physical-chemical properties.

ADDITIONAL RESOURCES

Review of Organic Functional Groups, Fifth Edition includes additional resources for both instructors and students.

Instructors

Approved adopting instructors will be given access to the following additional re-sources, which are available on the book's companion website at thePoint.lww.com/LemkeReview5e:

- PowerPoint slides
- An image bank of all the figures and tables in the book

Students

Students who have purchased *Review of Organic Functional Groups*, Fifth Edition have access to the following additional resources, via both an in-book CD-ROM and the book's companion website at thePoint.lww.com/LemkeReview5e:

- Problem sets corresponding to each of the organic functional groups (Chapters 2–17): Each problem set is followed by answers to the questions and a detailed discussion explaining the process leading to the answers. If you do not understand an answer or the process leading to the answer, re-turn to the appropriate section of the book and review that section again.
- Answers to the case studies found in the book.

In addition, purchasers of the text can access the searchable Full Text On-line by going to the *Review of Organic Functional Groups*, Fifth Edition website at thePoint.lww.com/LemkeReview5e. See the inside front cover of this text for more details, including the passcode you will need to gain access to the website.

ACKNOWLEDGMENTS

This book would not have been possible without the encouragement and input of colleagues and students. The idea for the text originated from a late-night discus-sion at a medicinal chemistry symposium and began as a series of tapes and slides that students were expected to review on their own time. A set of notes taken by students from the audiovisual presentations led to the initial development of a writ-ten manuscript which, with support from the SmithKline Corporation and the University of Houston College of Pharmacy, finally produced the first desktop copies of the book. In 1983, Lea & Febiger agreed to take a chance and published the first edition of this book, which has grown in size and quality over the years. The real joy comes from students, some of whom are now my colleagues, who in-formally tell me of the benefits they have gained from this book.

I want to acknowledge Drs. Victoria Roche and Sandy Zito, who have brought creativity, enthusiasm, and helpful suggestions in addition to their case studies to this edition of the book. I also want to thank the excellent staff, past and present, at LWW who have made this project seem more like an academic undertaking rather than a commercial process. Many of the staff members I have never met, but they do an excellent job of producing a quality product. I want to thank the staff that I have met and worked with over the years, which includes Matthew J. Hauber, David B. Troy, and Meredith Brittain. They have contributed greatly by keeping me on track and with encouraging words. Finally, a very special thanks goes out to my wife Pat, who puts up with me and the time spent working on the book, Flash, and PowerPoint presentations.

Contents

Preface iii

1   Water Solubility and Chemical Bonding 1
- Van der Waals Attraction (Forces) 2
- Dipole-Dipole Bonding (Hydrogen Bond) .2
- Ionic Attraction 3
- Ion-Dipole Bonding 4

2   Alkanes (C_nH_{2n+2}) 6

3   Alkenes (C_nH_{2n}) 11
- Cycloalkanes: Alkene Isomers 13

4   Aromatic Hydrocarbons 16

5   Haolgenated Hydrocarbons 19
- **Case Studies** 21

6   Alcohols 23
- **Case Studies** 27

7   Phenols 29
- **Case Studies** 34

8   Ethers and Thioethers 36
- Ethers 36
- Thioethers 38
- **Case Studies** 40

9   Aldehydes and Ketones 42
- **Case Studies** 47

10 Amines 49
- Amines—General 49
- Quaternary Ammonium Salts 58
- **Case Studies** 59

11 Carboxylic Acids 62
- **Case Studies** 70

12 Functional Derivatives of Carboxylic Acids 73
- Esters 73
- Amides 76
- Carbonates, Carbamates, and Ureas .79
- Amidines and Guanidines 81
- **Case Studies** 82

13 Sulfonic Acids and Sulfonamides .85
- Sulfonic Acids 85
- Sulfonamides 86
- **Case Studies** 87

14 Nitrogen Functional Groups 90
- Nitro Groups 90
- Nitrate Group 90
- Nitrite Group 91
- Oximes 92
- Hydrazone/Hydrazine/Hydrazide 92
- **Case Studies** 93

15 Heterocycles 96
- Three-Membered Ring Heterocycles .96
- Four-Membered Ring Heterocycles 99
- Five-Membered Ring Heterocycles 100
- Five-Membered Ring Heterocycles with Two or More
  Heteroatoms 105
- Six-Membered Ring Heterocycles 112
- Six-Membered Ring Heterocycles with Two Heteroatoms 114
- Saturated Six-Membered Ring Heterocycles 119
- Seven- and Eight-Membered Ring Heterocycles 120
- Bicyclic Heterocycles: Five-Membered Ring Plus
  Six-Membered Ring 120
- Bicyclic Heterocycles: Six-Membered Ring Plus
  Six-Membered Ring 125
- Bicyclic Heterocycles: Six-Membered Ring Plus
  Seven-Membered Ring 128
- Tricyclic Heterocycles 129
- **Case Studies** 130

16 Oligonucleotides and Nucleic Acids 133
- **Case Studies** 138

17 Proteins 141
  ▪ **Case Studies** 151

18 Predicting Water Solubility 153
  ▪ The Role of Chemical Bonding between Dissimilar
    Organic Functional Groups 153
  ▪ Empiric Method for Predicting Water Solubility 156
  ▪ Analytic Method for Calculating Water Solubility 160
  ▪ **Case Studies** 162

A Stereoisomerism—Asymmetric Molecules 164

B Acidity and Basicity 167
  ▪ Definitions of Acids and Bases 167
  ▪ Relative Strengths of Acids and Bases 169
  ▪ Reaction of an Acid with a Base in Water 171
  ▪ Acidic and Basic Organic Function Groups 173

C Drug Metabolism 176
  ▪ Metabolic Enzymes 176

D Learning Objectives 184

Glossary 187

Index 189

CHAPTER 1

Water Solubility and Chemical Bonding

At the outset, several definitions relating to organic compounds need to be discussed.

For our purposes, we will assume that an organic molecule will dissolve either in water or in a nonaqueous lipid solvent; that is, the organic molecule will not remain undissolved at the interphase of water and a lipid solvent. If a molecule dissolves fully or partially in water, it is said to be hydrophilic or to have hydrophilic character. The word "hydrophilic" is derived from "hydro," referring to water, and "philic," meaning loving or attracting. A substance that is hydrophilic may also be referred to, in a negative sense, as lipophobic. "Phobic" means fearing or hating, and thus lipophobic means lipid-hating, which therefore suggests that the chemical is water-loving.

If an organic molecule dissolves fully or partially in a nonaqueous or lipid solvent, the molecule is said to be lipophilic or to have lipophilic character. The term "lipophilic" or "lipid-loving" is synonymous with hydrophobic or water-hating, and these terms may be used interchangeably.

Hydrophilic	water-loving
Lipophobic	lipid-hating
Lipophilic	lipid-loving
Hydrophobic	water-hating

Water and lipid solubility are essential characteristics of a drug. For a drug to leave the gastrointestinal (GI) tract, it must pass through the lipid membrane of the GI tract. The drug will then enter the blood stream that is composed primarily of water. The drug can then be distributed throughout the body ultimately reaching the target cells on which or in which it is expected to act. To enter the cell the drug must again penetrate a lipid membrane and enter the aqueous intracellular fluid or cytosol. To leave the body, similar membranes and fluids must be traversed finally exiting the body through the kidney in aqueous urine or into the GI tract in biliary fluids. Thus, it should be recognized that aqueous and lipid solubility is essential for drug action.

To predict whether a chemical will dissolve in water or a lipid solvent, it must be determined whether the molecule and its functional groups can bond to water or the lipid solvent molecules. THIS IS THE KEY TO SOLUBILITY. If a molecule, through its functional groups, can bond to water, it will show some degree of water solubility. If, on the other hand, a molecule cannot bond to water, but instead bonds to the molecules of a lipid solvent, it will be water-insoluble or lipid-soluble. Our goal is therefore to determine to what extent a molecule can or cannot bond to water. To do this, we must define the types of intermolecular bonding that can occur between molecules.

What are the types of intermolecular bonds?

VAN DER WAALS ATTRACTION (FORCES)

The weakest type of interaction is electrostatic in nature and is known as van der Waals attraction or van der Waals forces. This type of attraction occurs between the nonpolar portion of two molecules and is brought about by a mutual distortion of electron clouds making up the covalent bonds (Fig. 1-1). This attraction is also referred to as the induced dipole-induced dipole attraction. In addition to being weak, it is temperature-dependent, being important at low temperatures and of little significance at high temperatures. The attraction occurs only over a short distance, thus requiring a tight packing of molecules. Steric factors, such as molecular branching, strongly influence van der Waals attraction. This type of chemical force is most prevalent in the hydrocarbon portion of organic molecules (aliphatic, alkene, aromatic systems). Van der Waals forces are approximately 0.5 to 1.0 kcal/mole for each atom involved. Van der Waals bonds are found in lipophilic solvents but are of little importance in water.

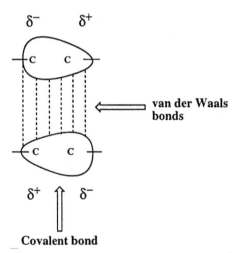

FIGURE 1-1. Van der Waals attraction resulting from distortion of covalent bonds.

DIPOLE-DIPOLE BONDING (HYDROGEN BOND)

A stronger and important form of chemical bonding is the dipole-dipole bond, a specific example of which is the hydrogen bond (Fig. 1-2). A dipole results from the unequal sharing of a pair of electrons making up a covalent bond. This occurs when the two atoms making up the covalent bond differ significantly in electronegativity. A partial ionic character develops in this portion of the molecule, leading to a permanent dipole, with the compound being described as a polar compound. The

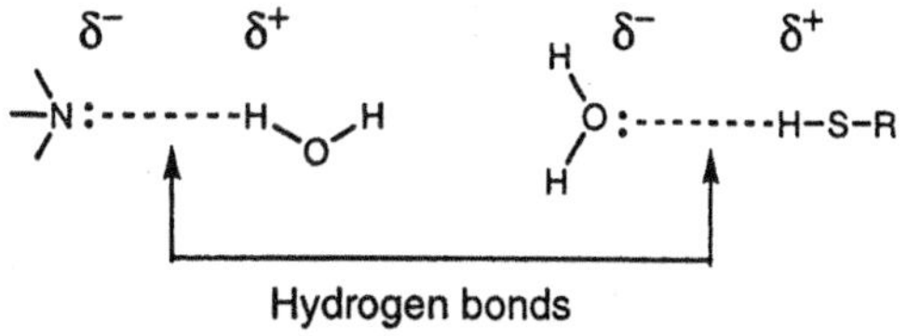

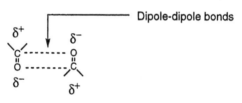

Hydrogen bonds

FIGURE 1-2. Hydrogen bonding of an amine to water and a thiol to water.

dipole-dipole attraction between two polar molecules arises from the negative end of one dipole being electrostatically attracted to the positive end of the second dipole. The hydrogen bond can occur when at least one dipole contains an electropositive hydrogen (e.g., a hydrogen covalently bonded to an electronegative atom such as oxygen, sulfur, nitrogen, or selenium), which in turn is attracted to a region of high electron density. Atoms with high electron densities are those with unshared pairs of electrons such as amine nitrogens, ether or alcohol oxygens, and thioether or thiol sulfurs. While hydrogen bonding is an example of dipole-dipole bonding, not all dipole-dipole bonding is hydrogen bonding (Fig. 1-3). Water, the

Dipole-dipole bonds

FIGURE 1-3. Dipole-dipole bonding between two ketone molecules.

important pharmaceutical solvent, is a good example of an hydrogen-bonding solvent. The ability of water to hydrogen bond accounts for the unexpectedly high boiling point of water as well as the characteristic dissolving properties of water. The hydrogen bond depends on temperature and distance. The energy of hydrogen bonding is 1.0 to 10.0 kcal/mole for each interaction.

IONIC ATTRACTION

A third type of bonding is the ionic attraction found quite commonly in inorganic molecules and salts of organic molecules. Ionic bonding results from the attraction of a negative atom for a positive atom (Fig. 1-4). The ionic bond involves a

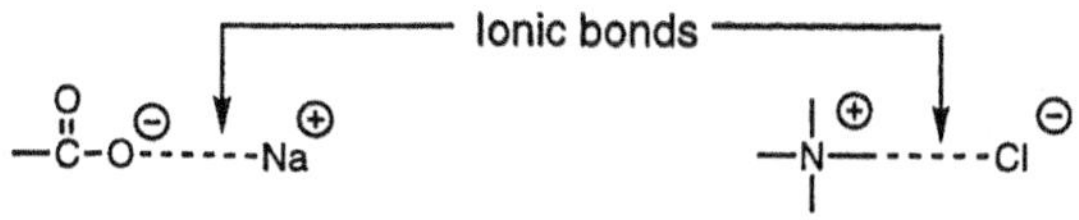

Ionic bonds

FIGURE 1-4. Ionic bonding found in salts of organic compounds.

somewhat stronger attractive force of 5 kcal/mole or more and is least affected by
temperature and distance.

ION-DIPOLE BONDING

Probably one of the most important chemical bonds involved in organic salts dissolving in water is the ion-dipole bond (Fig. 1-5). This bond occurs between an ion,

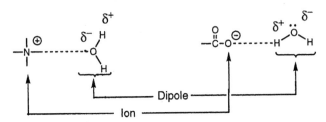

FIGURE 1-5. Ion-dipole bonding of a cationic amine to water and anionic
carboxylic acid to water.

either cation or anion, and a formal dipole, such as is found in water. The following two types of interactions may exist:

1. A cation will show bonding to a region of high electron density in a dipole
   (e.g., the oxygen atom in water).
2. An anion will bond to an electron-deficient region in a dipole (e.g., the
   hydrogen atom in water).

Ion-dipole bonding is a strong attraction that is relatively insensitive to temperature or distance. When an organic compound with basic properties (e.g., an amine)
is added to an aqueous acidic medium (pH below 7.0), the compound may form an
ionic salt that, if dissociable, will have enhanced water solubility owing to ion-dipole
bonding. Likewise, when an organic compound with acidic properties (e.g., carboxylic acids, phenols, unsubstituted or monosubstituted sulfonamides and unsubstituted imides) is added to an aqueous basic medium (pH above 7.0), the compound
may form an ionic salt that, if dissociable, will have enhanced water solubility owing
to ion-dipole bonding. Both of these examples are shown in Fig. 1-5.

Water is an important solvent from both a pharmaceutical and a biologic standpoint. Therefore, when looking at any drug from a structural viewpoint, it is important to know whether the drug will dissolve in water. To predict water solubility, one
must weigh the number and strength of hydrophilic groups in a molecule against the
lipophilic groups present. If a molecule has a large amount of water-loving character, by interacting with water through hydrogen bonding or ion-dipole attraction, it
would be expected to dissolve in water. If a molecule is deficient in hydrophilic
groups but instead has a lipophilic portion capable of van der Waals attraction, then
the molecule will most likely dissolve in a nonaqueous or lipophilic medium.

In reviewing the functional groups in organic chemistry, an attempt will be
made to identify the lipophilic or hydrophilic character of each functional group.

Knowing the character of each functional group in a drug will then allow an intelligent prediction of the overall solubility of the molecule by weighing the importance of each type of interaction. This book is organized in such a way that each functional group is discussed individually. Yet, when dealing with a drug molecule, the student will usually find a polyfunctional molecule. The ultimate goal is that the student should be able to predict the solubility of actual drugs in water, aqueous acidic media, and aqueous basic media. Therefore, to use this book correctly and to prepare yourself for the typical complex drug molecules, it is recommended that you read through Chapter 18 after studying each functional group. This will help you put each functional group into perspective with respect to polyfunctional molecules.

CATION-π BONDING

An unusual type of chemical bond is the cation-π bond. This electrostatic chemical bond exists between an electron-rich π system, such as that found in an aromatic ring, and a cation. The cation can be a metal (Li^+, Na^+, K^+) or an organic ammonium salt. The strength of the bond is similar to that

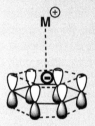

of the hydrogen bond and is effected by the nature of the cation and substitutions on the aromatic ring (groups that increase the electron density within the aromatic ring increase the strength of the bond). Recent studies have suggested that the cation-π bond is important for molecular recognition between cationic ligands and biologic receptors.

Cation-π recognition bonds between a tryptophan residue in the acetylcholine receptor and the ligands acetylcholine and nicotine.

Alkanes (C_nH_{2n+2})

2

■ **NOMENCLATURE.** The nomenclature of the alkanes may be either common or official nomenclature. The common nomenclature begins with the simplest system, methane, and proceeds to ethane, propane, butane, and so forth (Fig. 2-1). The "-ane" suffix indicates that the molecule is an alkane. This nomenclature works quite well until isomeric forms of the molecule appear (e.g., molecules with the same empirical formulas but different structural formulas). In butane, there are only two ways to put the molecule together, but as we consider larger molecules, many isomers are possible, and the nomenclature becomes unwieldy. Thus, a more systematic form of nomenclature is necessary. The IUPAC (International Union of Pure and Applied Chemistry) nomenclature is the official nomenclature.

IUPAC nomenclature requires that one find the longest continuous alkane chain. The name of this alkane chain becomes the base name. The chain is then numbered so as to provide the lowest possible numbers to the substituents. The number followed by the name of each substituent then precedes the base name of the straight-chain alkane. An example of naming an alkane according to IUPAC nomenclature is shown in Figure 2-2. The longest continuous chain is eight carbons.

This chain can be numbered from either end. Numbering left to right results in substituents at positions 2 (methyl), 5 (ethyl), and 7 (methyl). The name of this compound would be 5-ethyl-2,7-dimethyloctane. Numbering from right to left gives alkane substituents at the 2, 4, and 7 positions. This compound would be 4-ethyl-2, 7-dimethyloctane. To determine which way to number, add the numbers that correspond to the substituent locations and choose the direction that gives the lowest sum. From left to right, one has 2 + 5 + 7, which equals 14. When numbering from right to left, one has 2 + 4 + 7, which equals 13. Therefore, the correct numbering system

Structure	Common name
CH_4	Methane
CH_3-CH_3	Ethane
$CH_3-CH_2-CH_3$	Propane
$CH_3-CH_2-CH_2-CH_3$	*n*-Butane
$CH_3-\underset{\underset{CH_3}{\vert}}{CH}-CH_3$	*iso*-Butane

FIGURE 2-1. Common alkane nomenclature.

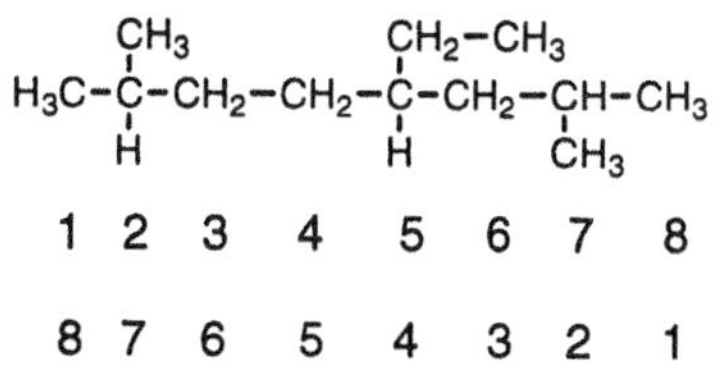

$$\begin{array}{c}
\qquad\quad CH_3 \qquad\qquad CH_2-CH_3 \\
H_3C-\underset{\underset{H}{|}}{C}-CH_2-CH_2-\underset{\underset{H}{|}}{C}-CH_2-\underset{\underset{CH_3}{|}}{CH}-CH_3
\end{array}$$

1 2 3 4 5 6 7 8

8 7 6 5 4 3 2 1

FIGURE 2-2. 4-Ethyl-2,7-dimethyloctane.

is from right to left, giving 4-ethyl-2,7-dimethyloctane. It should be noted that there is a convention for ordering the names of the substituents. The substituents are arranged in alphabetical order and appear before the base name of the molecule. Thus, ethyl precedes methyl. The number of groups present, in this case two methyls ("dimethyl") is not considered in this alphabetical arrangement.

When viewing complex drug molecules, the student will be expected to identify alkane portions of the drug and label these portions as alkanes using the generic nomenclature for such a functional group.

▪ **PHYSICAL-CHEMICAL PROPERTIES.** We wish to consider the following questions: Are alkanes going to be water-soluble, and can water solubility or the lack of it be explained? The physical-chemical properties of alkanes are readily understandable from the previous discussion of chemical bonding. These compounds are unable to undergo hydrogen bonding, ionic bonding, or ion-dipole bonding. The only inter-molecular bonding possible with these compounds is the weak van der Waals at-traction. For the smaller molecules with one to four carbon atoms, this bonding is not strong enough to hold the molecules together at room temperature, with the result that the lower-member alkanes are gases. For the larger molecules with 5 to 20 carbon atoms, the induced dipole-induced dipole interactions can occur, and the energy required to break the increased amount of bonding is more than is avail-able at room temperature. The result is that the 5- to 20-carbon atom alkanes are liquids. One can see from Table 2-1 that the boiling point increases consistently as more van der Waals bonding occurs.

Table 2-1. BOILING POINTS OF COMMON ALKANES

ALKANE	BOILING POINT (°C)
Propane	−42.0
n-Butane	−0.5
n-Pentane	36.1
n-Hexane	69.0
n-Heptane	98.4
n-Octane	126.0

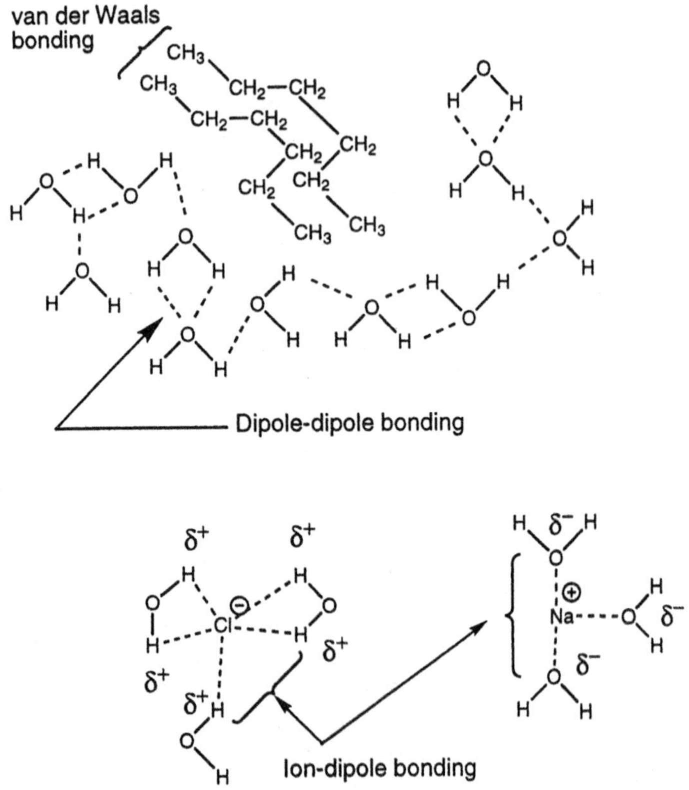

FIGURE 2-3. Diagram of *n*-hexane's lack of solubility in water and the solubility of sodium chloride in water through ion-dipole bonding.

The effects of adding an alkane to water are depicted in Figure 2-3. Water is an ordered medium with a considerable amount of inter-molecular bonding, indicated by its high boiling point (i.e., high in respect to its molecular weight). To dissolve in or to mix with water, foreign atoms must break into this lattice. Sodium chloride (table salt), which is quite water-soluble, is an example of a molecule capable of this. An alkane cannot break into the water lattice since it cannot bond to water. Ion-dipole interaction, which is possible for sodium chloride, is not possible for the alkane. Ionic bonding and hydrogen bonding between water and the alkane also are not possible. Van der Waals bonding between alkane and alkane is relatively strong, with little or no van der Waals attraction between the water and the alkane. The net result is that the alkane separates out and is immiscible in water. Alkanes will dissolve in a lipid solvent or oil layer. The term "lipid," "fat," or "oil," defined from the standpoint of solubility, means a water-immiscible or water-insoluble material. Lipid solvents are rich in alkane groups; therefore, it is not surprising that alkanes are soluble in lipid layers, since induced dipole-induced dipole bonding will be abundant. If an alkane has a choice between remaining in an aqueous area or moving to a lipid area, it will move to the lipid area. In chemistry, this means that if n-heptane is placed in a separatory funnel containing water and decane, the n-heptane will partition into the decane. This movement of alkanes also occurs in biologic systems and is best represented by the general anesthetic alkanes and their rapid partitioning into the lipid portion of the brain, while at the same time they have poor affinity for the aqueous blood. This concept will be discussed in detail in courses in medicinal chemistry.

Another property that should be mentioned is chemical stability. In the case of alkanes, one is dealing with a stable compound. For our purposes, these compounds are to be considered chemically inert to the conditions met "on the shelf"—namely, air, light, aqueous acid or base, and heat.

A final physical-chemical property that may be encountered in branched-chain alkanes is seen when a carbon atom is substituted with four different substituents (Fig. 2-4). Such a molecule is said to be asymmetric (i.e., without a plane or point

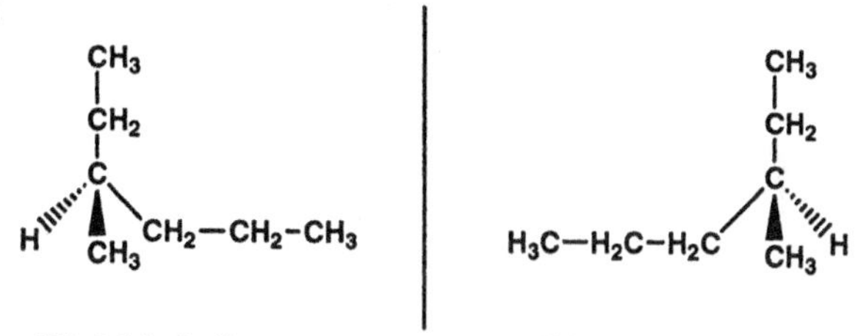

(S)-3-Methylhexane　　　　(R)-3-Methylhexane

FIGURE 2-4. Structures of (S)-3-methylhexane and its mirror image, (R)-3-methylhexane.

of symmetry) and is referred to as a chiral molecule. Chirality in a molecule means that the molecule exists as two stereoisomers, which are nonsuperimposable mirror images of each other, as shown in Figure 2-4. These stereoisomers are referred to as enantiomeric forms of the molecule and possess the same physical and chemical properties with the exception of the direction that each isomer will rotate plane polarized light. One isomer will rotate plane polarized light to the left while the other isomer will rotate the light to the right (both to the same degree). In addition, chirality in a molecule usually leads to significant biological differences in biologically active molecules. The topic of stereoisomerism is reviewed briefly in Appendix A.

■ **METABOLISM.** The alkane functional group is relatively nonreactive in vivo and will be excreted from the body unchanged. Although the student should consider the alkanes themselves as nonreactive and the alkane portions of a drug as nonreactive, several notable exceptions will be emphasized in the medicinal chemistry courses, and they should be learned as exceptions. Two such exceptions are shown in Figure 2-5. When metabolism does occur, it is commonly an oxidation reaction catalyzed by a cytochrome P450 isoform (CYP450) previously known as

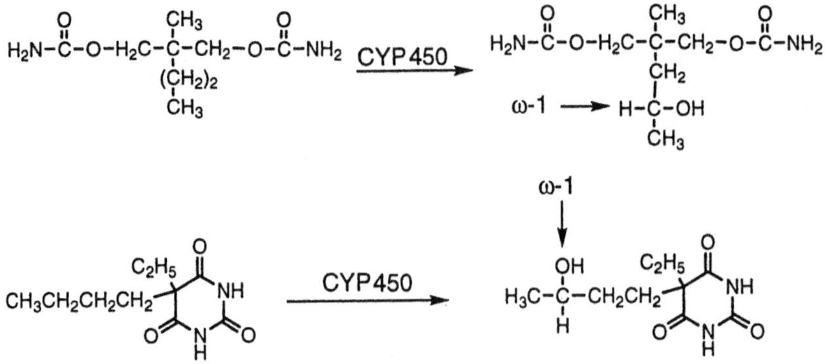

FIGURE 2-5. Metabolism of meprobamate and butylbarbital.

mixed-function oxidase enzymes, and in most cases it occurs at the end of the hydrocarbon, the omega carbon, or adjacent to the final carbon at the omega-minus-one carbon, as shown. For additional discussion of the metabolic process see Appendix C, Metabolism.

Alkenes (C_nH_{2n})

3

■ **NOMENCLATURE.** The common nomenclature for the alkenes uses the radical name representing the total number of carbons present and the suffix "-ene," which indicates the presence of a double bond (Fig. 3-1). This type of nomenclature becomes awkward for branched-chain alkenes, and the official IUPAC nomenclature becomes useful. With IUPAC nomenclature, the longest continuous chain containing the double bond is chosen and is given a base name that corresponds to the alkane of that length. As indicated in Figure 3-2, the longest chain has seven carbons and is therefore a heptane derivative. The chain is numbered so as to assign the lowest possible number to the double bond. In numbering left to right, the double bond is at the 3 position, which is preferred, rather than numbering right to left, which would put the double bond at the 4 position. With the molecule correctly numbered, the final step in naming the compound consists of naming and numbering the alkyl radicals, followed by the location of the double bond and the alkane name, in which the "-ane" is dropped

Structure	Common name
$CH_2=CH_2$	Ethylene
$CH_2=CH-CH_3$	Propylene
$CH_2=CH-CH_2-CH_3$	1-Butylene
$CH_2=\underset{\underset{CH_3}{\vert}}{C}-CH_3$	*iso*-Butylene

FIGURE 3-1. Common alkene nomenclature.

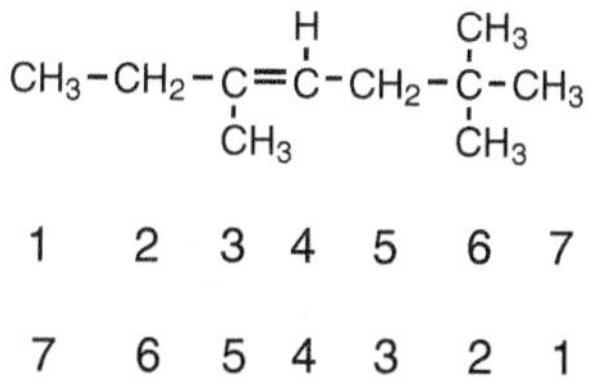

$$CH_3-CH_2-\underset{\underset{CH_3}{\vert}}{C}=\overset{\overset{H}{\vert}}{C}-CH_2-\underset{\underset{CH_3}{\vert}}{\overset{\overset{CH_3}{\vert}}{C}}-CH_3$$

1   2   3   4   5   6   7

7   6   5   4   3   2   1

FIGURE 3-2. 3,6,6-Trimethyl-3-heptene.

and replaced with the "-ene." In the example, the correct name would be 3,6,6-trimethyl-3 (the location of the double bond) hept (seven carbons) ene (meaning an alkene).

In complex molecules, the student will be expected to identify the alkene and label it as such. The student should then associate the appropriate physical-chemical and metabolic properties to the alkene functional group.

The introduction of a double bond into a molecule also raises the possibility of geometric isomers. Isomers are compounds with the same empirical formula but a different structural formula. If the difference in structural formulas comes from lack of free rotation around a bond, this is referred to as a geometric isomer. 2-Butene may exist as a *trans*-2-butene or *cis*-2-butene, which are examples of geometric isomers (Fig. 3-3). The "E,Z" nomenclature has been instituted to deal with

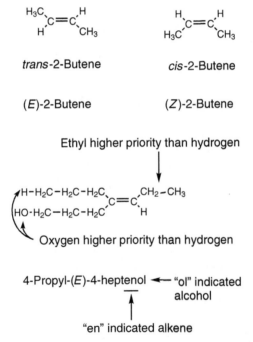

FIGURE 3-3. Examples of E,Z nomenclature for naming alkenes.

tri- and tetra-substituted alkenes, which cannot be readily named by cis/trans nomenclature. The "E" is taken from the German word *entgegen*, which means opposite, and the "Z" from *zusammen*, meaning together. Using a series of priority rules, if the two substituents of highest priority are on the same side of the π bond, the configuration of Z is assigned, whereas if the two high-priority groups are on opposite sides, the E configuration is used. In the example in Figure 3-2, the correct nomenclature becomes (E)-3,6,6-trimethyl-3-heptene.

▪ **PHYSICAL-CHEMICAL PROPERTIES.** The physical properties of the alkenes are similar to those of the alkanes. The lower members, having two through four carbon atoms, are gases at room temperature. Alkenes with five carbon atoms or more are liquids with increasing boiling points corresponding to increases in molecular weight. The weak intermolecular interaction that accounts for the low boiling point is again of the induced dipole-induced dipole type. Recognizing what type of intermolecular interaction is possible also allows a prediction of nonaqueous versus aqueous solubility. Since alkenes cannot hydrogen bond and have a weak permanent dipole, they cannot dissolve in the aqueous layer. Alkenes will dissolve in nonpolar solvents such as lipids, fats, or oil layers. Therefore, the physical properties of alkenes parallel those of the alkanes. When the chemical properties are considered, a departure from similarity to the alkane is found. The multiple bond gives the molecule a reactive site. From a pharmaceutical standpoint, alkenes are prone to oxidation, leading to peroxide or hydroperoxide formation (Fig. 3-4). Such a reaction, if it occurs, is more common with gaseous alkenes. Peroxides are quite unstable and may explode. In addition, alkenes, especially the volatile members, are quite flammable and may explode in the presence of oxygen and a spark.

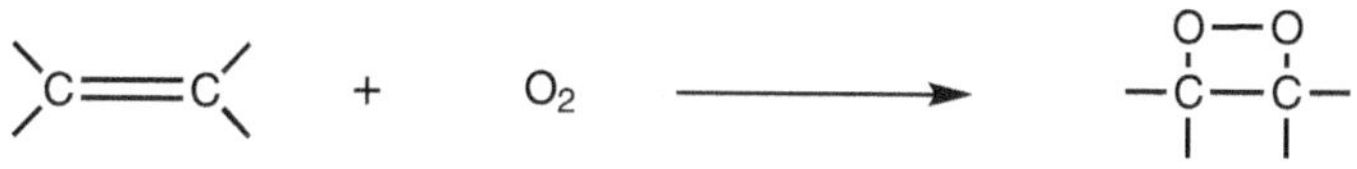

FIGURE 3-4. Oxidation of an alkene with molecular oxygen leading to a peroxide.

▪ **METABOLISM.** Metabolism of the alkenes, as with the previously discussed alkanes, is not common. For our purposes, the alkene functional group should be considered metabolically stable. While alkene-containing drugs are usually stable in the body, the alkene functional groups of several body metabolites serve as centers of reaction (Fig. 3-5). The unsaturated fatty acids add water to give alcohols. A cytochrome P450 oxidase attacks the alkene functional group in squalene to give an epoxide during the biosynthesis of steroids. A peroxide intermediate is formed from eicosatrienoate, a triene, during prostaglandin biosynthesis, and during saturated fatty acid synthesis, alkenes are reduced in vivo. You should be familiar, therefore, with these possible reactions of the alkene functional group and should not be surprised if an alkene-containing drug is metabolized.

CYCLOALKANES: ALKENE ISOMERS

Before leaving the topic of alkenes, a group of compounds that are isomeric to the alkenes should be mentioned. The cycloalkanes have the same empirical formula, C_nH_{2n}, as the alkenes but possess a different structural formula and are therefore isomeric. Three important members of this class are cyclopropane, cyclopentane, and cyclohexane (Fig. 3-6). Cyclopropane acts chemically like propene, while

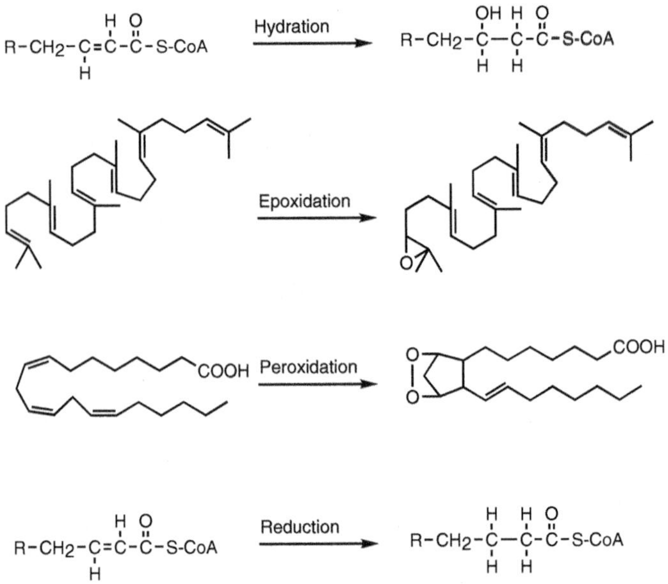

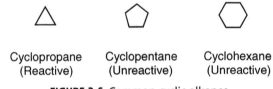

$$R-CH_2-C{=}C-\overset{O}{\overset{\|}{C}}-S\text{-}CoA \xrightarrow{\text{Hydration}} R-CH_2-\overset{OH}{\underset{H}{\overset{|}{C}}}-\overset{H}{\underset{H}{\overset{|}{C}}}-\overset{O}{\overset{\|}{C}}-S\text{-}CoA$$

Epoxidation

COOH   Peroxidation

$$R-CH_2-C{=}C-\overset{O}{\overset{\|}{C}}-S\text{-}CoA \xrightarrow{\text{Reduction}} R-CH_2-\overset{H}{\underset{H}{\overset{|}{C}}}-\overset{H}{\underset{H}{\overset{|}{C}}}-\overset{O}{\overset{\|}{C}}-S\text{-}CoA$$

FIGURE 3-5. Metabolic reactions of alkene-containing molecules.

Cyclopropane   Cyclopentane   Cyclohexane
(Reactive)   (Unreactive)   (Unreactive)

FIGURE 3-6. Common cyclic alkanes.

cyclopentane and cyclohexane are chemically inert, much like the alkanes. All three compounds are lipid-soluble and quite flammable. The latter two ring systems are common to many drug molecules.

Similar to the alkenes, the cycloalkanes do not show free rotation around the carbon-carbon bonds of the cycloalkane and as a result have the potential of geometric isomers. With polysubstituted cycloalkanes *cis* and *trans* isomers exist, resulting in compounds with different physical-chemical properties. An added characteristic of cycloalkanes with six or more carbons (less so with cyclopentane) is the ability of the molecule to exist in different conformational forms or isomers. While conformational isomers of a molecule (i.e., the way the molecule stands in space) do not change the physical-chemical properties of a molecule, nor are these isomers separable, conformational isomers of a molecule may affect the way that

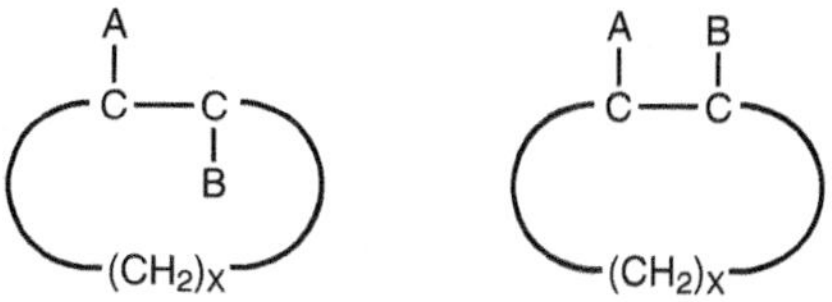

trans isomer   cis isomer

the molecule is drawn. As an example, *trans*-1,2-dimethylcyclohexane has a high energy conformation drawn with the methyl groups in their axial conformation and a low energy conformation with the methyls in the equatorial conformation (Fig. 3-7). The significance of conformational isomers of a molecule becomes important when considering drug-receptor interactions and will be discussed in medicinal chemistry courses.

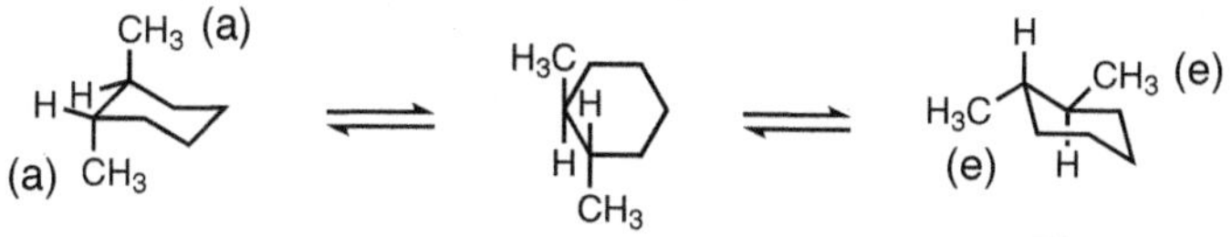

axial *trans*-1,2-dimethyl-
cyclohexane
(high energy conformation)

equatorial *trans*-1,2-dimethyl-
cyclohexane
(low energy conformation)

[(a) = axial, (e) = equatorial]

FIGURE 3-7. Examples of the conformational isomers of *trans*-1,2-dimethylcyclohexane.

Aromatic Hydrocarbons

CHAPTER

4

■ **NOMENCLATURE.** Another class of hydrocarbons, shown in Figure 4-1, is the aromatic hydrocarbons. In aromatic nomenclature, a single name is used for the aromatic nucleus. Several of the most common nuclei have been shown, along with their official name and numbering system.

■ **PHYSICAL-CHEMICAL PROPERTIES.** At first glance, it might be thought that the aromatic hydrocarbons are nothing more than cyclic alkenes, but this is not the case. Remember that aromatic compounds do not have isolated single and double bonds; instead, they have a cloud of electrons above and below the ring. This is a cloud of delocalized electrons that are not as readily available as the electrons in the alkenes. The aromatic systems are therefore not as prone to the chemical reactions that affect alkenes.

Formation of peroxides, a potentially serious pharmaceutical problem with many alkenes, is not considered a problem with the aromatic hydrocarbons. The typical reaction of the aromatic systems is the electrophilic reaction. In the electrophilic reaction, the electrophile, the electron-loving, positively charged species, attacks the electron-dense cloud of the aromatic ring. There is one significant electrophilic reaction that occurs only in biologic systems, and this is known as hydroxylation. This

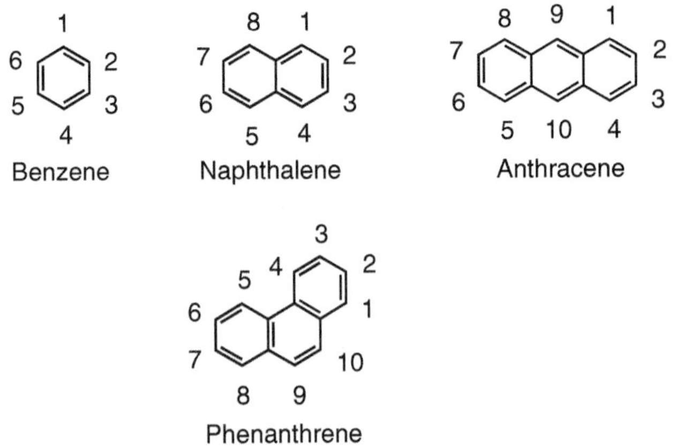

FIGURE 4-1. Aromatic nomenclature and numbering of common aromatic rings.

reaction is quite important during drug metabolism but does not occur in vitro. Aromatic hydrocarbons are quite stable on the shelf. These hydrocarbons, like other hydrocarbons, are lipophilic and flammable. Because of their high electron density and flat nature, however, aromatic hydrocarbons show a somewhat stronger capacity to bond through van der Waals attraction. Aromatic rings appear to play a significant role in the binding of a drug to biologic proteins, as will be seen in courses on medicinal chemistry.

■ **METABOLISM.** As already mentioned, aromatic rings are quite prone to oxidation in vivo or, more specifically, to aromatic hydroxylation. This reaction is commonly catalyzed by several of the cytochrome P450 isoforms and may involve an initial epoxidation. In a few cases, this highly reactive epoxide has been isolated, but in most cases the epoxide rearranges to give the hydroxylation product, the phenol or dialcohol, as shown in Figure 4-2. The importance of this reaction is considerable.

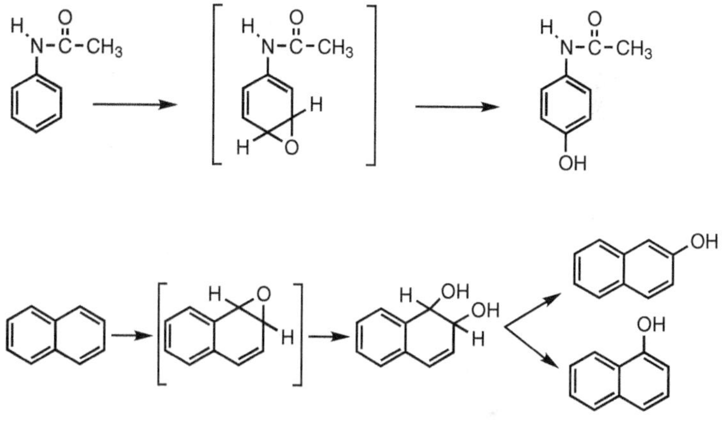

FIGURE 4-2. Aromatic hydroxylation catalyzed by cytochrome P450 (CYP 450).

Aromatic hydroxylation significantly increases the water solubility of the aromatic system (See Chapter 7, Phenols). In many cases this results in a rapid removal of the chemical from the body, while in a few cases hydroxylation may actually increase the activity of the drug. An area of considerable importance has been the study of the role of hydroxylation of aromatic hydrocarbons and its relationship to the carcinogenic properties of aromatic hydrocarbons. Evidence suggests that the intermediate epoxides are responsible for this carcinogenic effect.

As indicated, the phenols formed by aromatic hydroxylation may be eliminated as such from the body or may undergo a phase 2 conjugation, giving rise to a sulfate

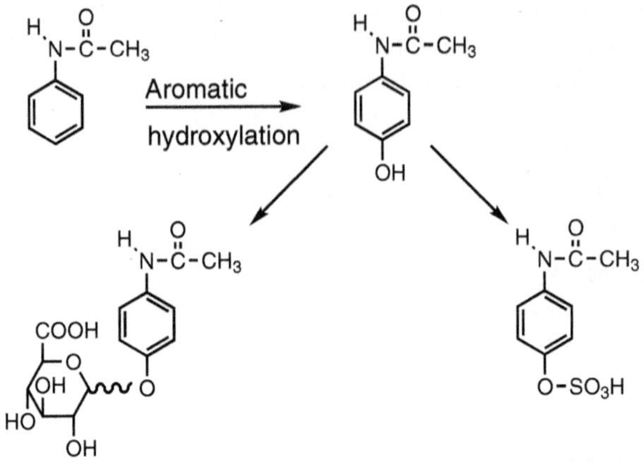

FIGURE 4-3. Phase 2 conjugation reaction of aromatic hydroxylation product.

conjugate or a glucuronide conjugate, as shown in Figure 4-3. These conjugates exhibit an even greater water solubility (see Appendix C, Metabolism for discussion of conjugation reactions).

Halogenated Hydrocarbons

5

■ **NOMENCLATURE.** The common nomenclature for mono-substituted halogenated hydrocarbons consists of the name of the alkyl radical followed by the name of the halogen atom. Examples of this nomenclature, along with the structures and names of several common polyhalogenated hydrocarbons, are shown in Figure 5-1.

This nomenclature again becomes complicated as the branching of the hydrocarbon chain increases, and one therefore uses IUPAC nomenclature. The IUPAC nomenclature requires choosing the longest continuous hydrocarbon chain, followed by numbering of the chain so as to assign the lowest number to the halide. The compound is then named as a haloalkane. This is illustrated in Figure 5-2 for 2-bromo-4-methylpentane.

■ **PHYSICAL-CHEMICAL PROPERTIES.** The properties of the halogenated hydrocarbons differ somewhat from those of the hydrocarbons previously discussed. The monohaloalkanes have a permanent dipole owing to the strongly electronegative

Structure	Common name
CH_3-F	Methylfluoride
CH_3-CH_2-Cl	Ethylchloride
$CH_3-CH_2-CH_2-Br$	Propylbromide
$CH_3-CH_2-CH_2-CH_2-I$	*n*-Butyliodide
CH_2Cl_2	Methylene chloride
$CHCl_3$	Chloroform
CCl_4	Carbontetrachloride
$Cl-CH_2-CH_2-Cl$	Ethylene chloride

FIGURE 5-1. Common halogenated hydrocarbon nomenclature.

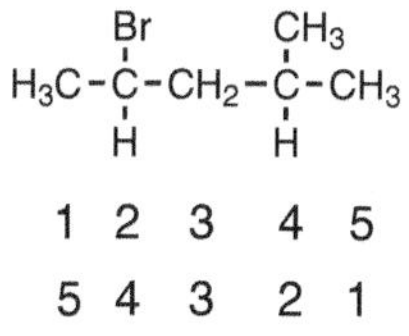

$$H_3C-\overset{\overset{\displaystyle Br}{|}}{\underset{\underset{\displaystyle H}{|}}{C}}-CH_2-\overset{\overset{\displaystyle CH_3}{|}}{\underset{\underset{\displaystyle H}{|}}{C}}-CH_3$$

1 2 3 4 5

5 4 3 2 1

FIGURE 5-2. 2-Bromo-4-methylpentane.

halide attached to the carbon. The permanent dipole does not guarantee dipole-dipole bonding, however. Although the halogen is rich in electron density, there is no region highly deficient in electrons, and intermolecular bonding is therefore weak and again depends on the van der Waals attraction. Since only van der Waals bonding is possible, these compounds have low boiling points and poor water solubility. The halogens covalently bound to carbon in general increase the lipophilic nature of the compounds to which they are bound. Another property of the halogenated hydrocarbons is a decrease in flammability with an increase in the number of halogens. In fact, carbon tetrachloride has been used in fire extinguishers. In general, these compounds are highly lipid-soluble and chemically nonreactive.

One important chemical reaction that methylene chloride, chloroform, and several other polyhalogenated compounds undergo is shown in Figure 5-3. Chloroform, in the presence of oxygen and heat, is converted to phosgene, a reactive and toxic chemical. To destroy any phosgene that may form in a bottle of chloroform, a small amount of alcohol is usually present. The alcohol reacts with the phosgene to give a nontoxic carbonate.

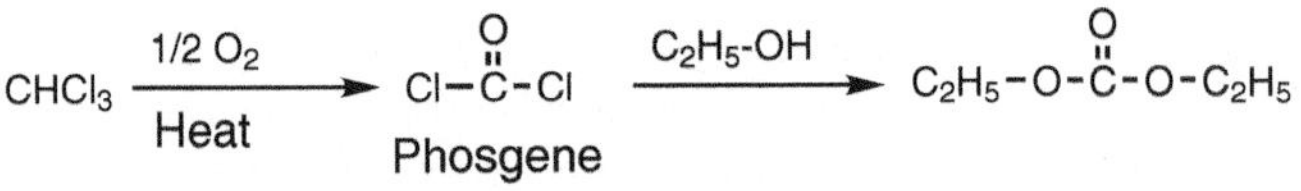

FIGURE 5-3. Oxidation of chloroform to phosgene.

It should be noted that this oxidative reaction is limited to volatile short-chain polyhalogenated compounds. A polyhalogenated carbon within a larger organic molecule will not undergo oxidative dehalogenation.

■ **METABOLISM.** The lack of chemical reactivity in vitro carries over to in vivo stability. In general, halogenated hydrocarbons are not readily metabolized and this is especially true of halogenated aromatic compounds. A notable exception to the stability of haloalkanes is seen with the halogenated general anesthetics. Oxidative dehydrohalogenation of these drugs is quite common and is catalyzed by cytochrome P450. The reaction requires at least one hydrogen (α-hydrogen) attached to the carbon containing the halogen and appears to be dependent on the stabilizing action of the adjacent halogen and its unshared pairs of electrons. The oxidation leads initially to a halohydrin, which then eliminates a hydrohalic acid (Fig. 5-4). Adjacent (gem) trihalo or dihalo carbon moieties increase the rate of this reaction. The reactive

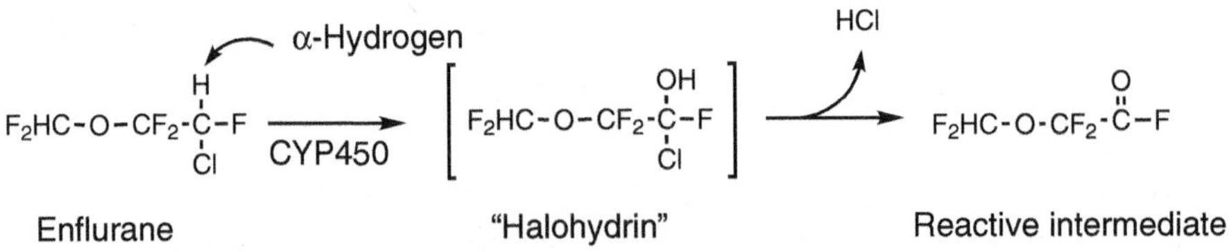

FIGURE 5-4. Metabolic oxidative dehydrohalogenation of enflurane.

intermediate formed following dehydrohalogenation is associated with both hepato-toxicity and nephrotoxicity. Since the halogenated hydrocarbons are quite lipid sol-uble, they are not readily excreted by the kidney and have prolonged biologic half-life, increasing the likelihood for systemic toxicity. This may also account for the potential carcinogenic properties of some halogenated hydrocarbons.

In summary, one significant property is common to all of the hydrocarbons, and that is the lack of ability to bond to water and thus the lipophilic or hydrophobic nature. SINCE ALL ORGANIC MOLECULES HAVE A HYDROCARBON PORTION, THIS PROPERTY WILL SHOW UP TO SOME EXTENT IN ALL MOLECULES. You will have to weigh the extent of influence of the lipophilic por-tion against the quantity of hydrophilic character to predict whether a molecule will dissolve in a nonaqueous medium or in water.

Note: Case Studies 5.1 and 5.2 incorporate information from Chapters 2 through 5 of this book.

Case Study 5.1

As the medicinal chemist of the drug design "dream team" at Lemke Pharmaceuticals, you are leading your group in the construction of a structure that will bind with high affinity to a novel binding site on the VEGF (vascular endothelial growth factor) protein. The goal is the development of a drug that will inhibit unwanted growth of new blood vessels, and be of use in the treat-ment of "wet" macular degeneration and cancer. The binding site has been mod-eled, and one specific area is known to be sterically restricted (e.g., a narrow channel within the protein) and lined with Ala, Trp, and Tyr residues. The mo-lecular region of your lead compound (known as lunamine) that will be interact-ing with this site is shown in the following figure as "R."

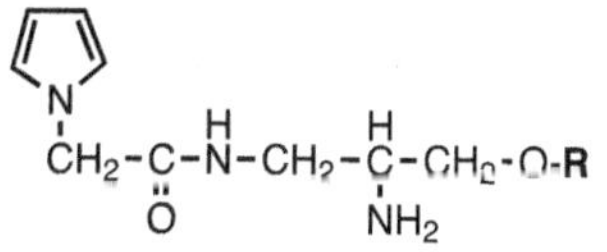

Lunamine (lead compound)

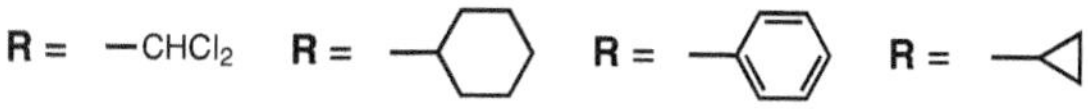

$$R = \quad -CHCl_2 \qquad R = \quad \bigcirc \qquad R = \quad \bigcirc \qquad R = \quad \triangleleft$$

| 1 | 2 | 3 | 4 |

Discuss the feasibility of each of the four candidates for this "R" substituent in light of the binding site restrictions, and make a recommendation to your syn-thetic team. Since nothing is ever truly perfect, identify one potential disadvan-tage to your recommendation.

Case Study 5.2

You are the night pharmacist in your local hospital and known for your interest and expertise in the chemical foundation of drug therapy. You receive a call from the burn unit dealing with a case of a young man who received third-degree burns on his face as a result of his practice of inhaling the aerosols used as propellants for electronic dusting while smoking cigarettes. The physician in charge tells you that he thought these dusting propellants were just "air in the can" and were harmless; however, he discovered that they contain one of a number of halogenated hydrocarbons and presents you with the following structures and asks you the following questions:

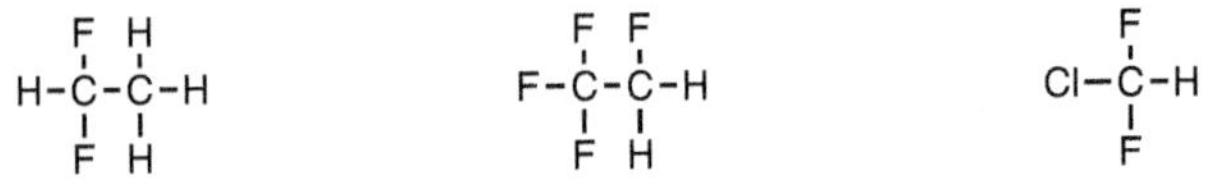

```
        F  H                 F  F                    F
        |  |                 |  |                    |
    H-C-C-H             F-C-C-H              Cl-C-H
        |  |                 |  |                    |
        F  H                 F  H                    F

 1,1-Difluoroethane  1,1,1,2-Tetrafluoroethane  Chlorodifluoromethane
      (DFE)                   (TFE)                    (CDF)
```

Halogenated hydrocarbons commonly used in aerosol dusting products.

1. What accounts for the volatility of the halogenated hydrocarbons?
2. Which of the possible halogenated hydrocarbons is the most flammable and therefore the propellant involved in this case?
3. Are there any metabolic issues that the physician should be aware of in treating this patient?

Alcohols

6

■ **NOMENCLATURE.** The common nomenclature of alcohols is to name the molecule as an "alcohol" preceded by the names of the hydrocarbon radical (Fig. 6-1). Methyl and ethyl alcohol are examples of primary alcohols, isopropyl alcohol is an example of a secondary alcohol, and tertiary butyl alcohol is an example of a tertiary alcohol. The primary, secondary, and tertiary designations given to an alcohol depend upon the number of carbons that are attached to the carbon that contains the OH group. The primary designation indicates that one carbon is attached to the carbon bearing the OH group; the secondary designation indicates that two carbons are attached; and the tertiary designation indicates that three carbons are attached.

Once again, the nomenclature becomes clumsy as the hydrocarbon portion branches, and the official IUPAC nomenclature must be used (see Fig. 6-1). The longest continuous chain that contains the hydroxyl group is chosen. The chain is then numbered to give the lowest number to the hydroxyl group. Other substituents, preceded by their numbered location, come first, followed by the location of the hydroxyl group, followed by the name of the alkane. To show that this is an alcohol, the "e" is dropped from the alkane name and replaced by "ol," the official sign of an alcohol.

It is essential that the student be able to identify an alcohol functional group within a complex molecule and assign primary, secondary, or tertiary designation to the group.

Structure	Common name	IUPAC name
CH_3-OH	Methyl alcohol (Wood alcohol)	Methanol
CH_3-CH_2-OH	Ethyl alcohol (Alcohol USP)	Ethanol
$CH_3-\underset{\underset{CH_3}{\mid}}{CH}-OH$	Isopropyl alcohol (Rubbing alcohol)	2-Propanol
$CH_3-\underset{\underset{CH_3}{\mid}}{\overset{\overset{CH_3}{\mid}}{C}}-OH$	*tert*-Butyl alcohol	2-Methyl-2-propanol

FIGURE 6-1. Common and IUPAC nomenclature for alcohols.

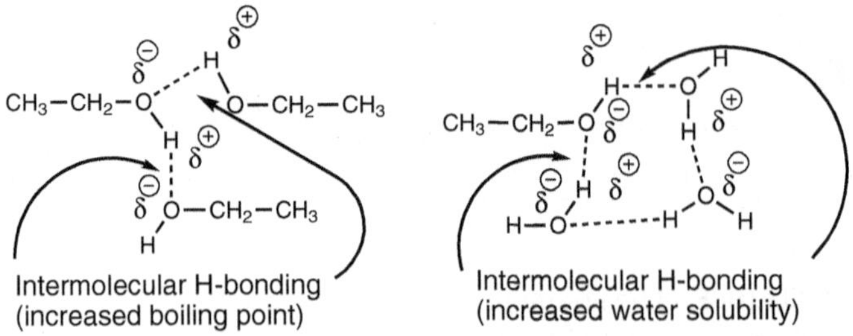

FIGURE 6-2. Examples of intermolecular hydrogen bonding (H-bonding) between molecules of ethanol and between ethanol and water.

■ **PHYSICAL-CHEMICAL PROPERTIES.** The properties of the alcohol offer a departure from the compounds that have been discussed previously. The OH group can participate in intermolecular hydrogen bonding (Fig. 6-2). Because of the electronegativity of the oxygen and the electropositive proton, a permanent dipole exists. The hydrogen attached to the oxygen is slightly positive in nature and the oxygen slightly negative. Remember, this is not a formal charge but simply an unequal sharing of the pair of electrons that make up the covalent bond. The intermolecular hydrogen bonding that is now possible between the alcohol molecules results in relatively high boiling points compared with their hydrocarbon counterparts (Table 6-1). Also important is the fact that the alcohol group can hydrogen bond to water (see Fig. 6-2). This means that it can break into the water lattice, with the result that the alcohol functional group promotes water solubility. The extent of water solubility for each alcohol will depend on the size of the hydrocarbon portion (see Table 6-1). C_1 through C_3 alcohols are miscible with water in all proportions. As the length of the hydrocarbon chain increases, the hydrophilic nature of the molecule decreases. The location of the hydroxyl radical also influences water solubility, although not as dramatically as chain length. A hydroxyl group

Table 6-1. BOILING POINTS AND WATER SOLUBILITY OF COMMON ALCOHOLS

	BOILING POINTS °C	SOLUBILITY (g/100g H_2O)
Methanol	65.5	∝
Ethanol	78.3	∝
1-Propanol	97.0	∝
2-Propanol	82.4	∝
1-Butanol	117.2	7.9
2-Butanol	99.5	12.5
1-Pentanol	137.3	2.3

centered in the molecule will have a greater potential for producing water solubility than a hydroxyl at the end of the straight chain. If a second hydroxyl is added, solubility is increased. An example of this is 1,5-pentanediol. It can be thought of as ethanol and propanol put together. Since both alcohols are quite water-soluble, it would be predicted that 1,5-pentanediol would also be quite water-soluble, and it is. It also follows that as the solubility of the alcohol in water decreases, the solubility of the alcohol in nonaqueous media increases. In summary, it can be said that an alcohol functional group has the ability to solubilize to the extent of 1% or greater an alkane chain of five or six carbon atoms.

Looking at the chemical reactivity of the alcohol, we find that from a pharmaceutical standpoint the alcohol functional group is a relatively stable unit. Remember, though, that in the presence of oxidizing agents, a primary alcohol will be oxidized to a carboxylic acid after passing through an intermediate aldehyde (Fig. 6-3). The secondary alcohols can be oxidized to a ketone, and a tertiary alcohol is stable to mild oxidation. The oxidation of an alcohol in vitro is not commonly encountered because of the limited number of oxidating agents used pharmaceutically.

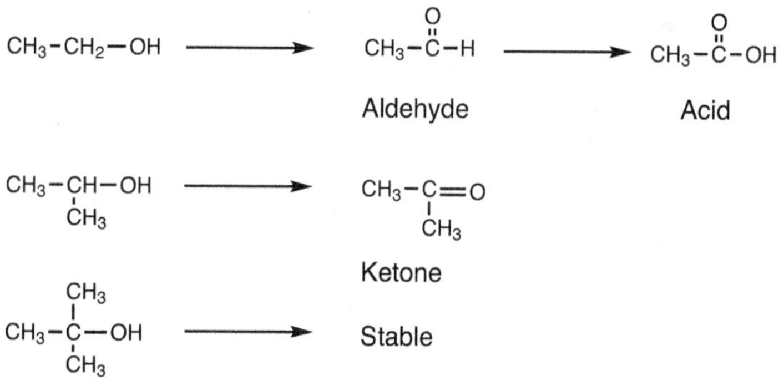

FIGURE 6-3. Oxidation of a primary and secondary alcohol by oxidizing agents (normally uncommon in pharmaceutical products).

▪ **METABOLISM.** Although the alcohol functional group is relatively stable in vitro, it is readily metabolized in the body by a variety of enzymes, most notably cytochrome P450 enzymes and alcohol dehydrogenase. Alcohol dehydrogenase, a NAD-specific enzyme, is the more common oxidizing enzyme. Both primary and secondary alcohols are prone to oxidation by oxidase enzymes, resulting in the formation of carboxylic acids or ketones, respectively (Fig. 6-4). This metabolism represents a phase 1 metabolism. The tertiary alcohols are stable to oxidase enzymes. Alcohols are also prone to phase 2 type metabolisms, the most common of which is glucuronidation reaction. This reaction consists of conjugation of an alcohol with activated glucuronic

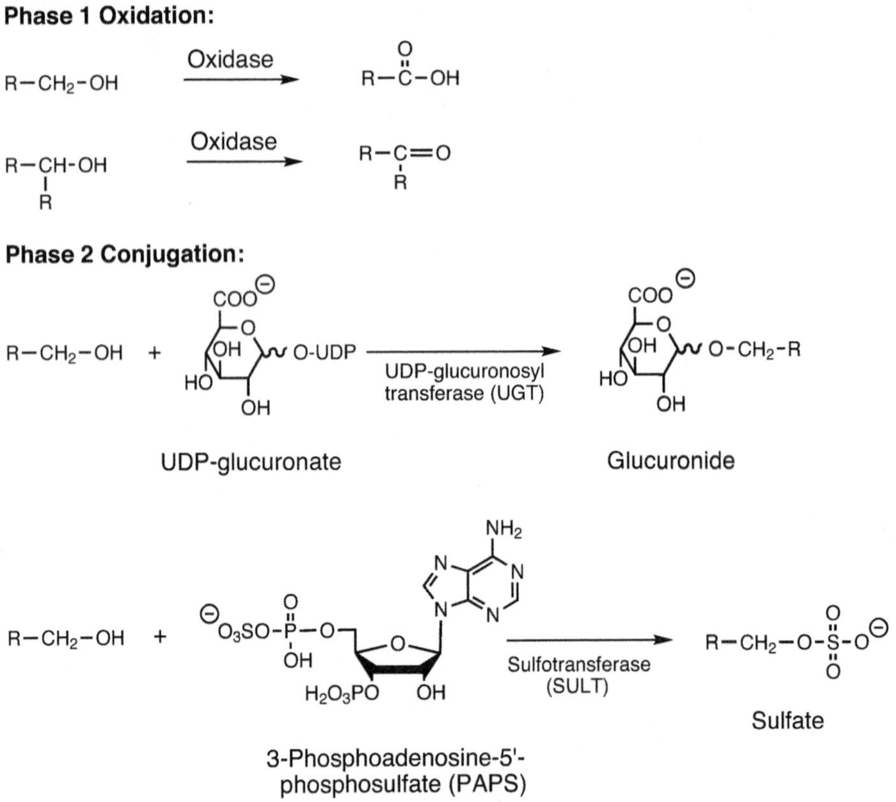

Phase 1 Oxidation:

$$R-CH_2-OH \xrightarrow{\text{Oxidase}} R-\overset{\overset{\displaystyle O}{\|}}{C}-OH$$

$$R-\underset{\underset{\displaystyle R}{|}}{CH}-OH \xrightarrow{\text{Oxidase}} R-\underset{\underset{\displaystyle R}{|}}{C}=O$$

Phase 2 Conjugation:

UDP-glucuronate   Glucuronide

3-Phosphoadenosine-5'-
phosphosulfate (PAPS)

FIGURE 6-4. Metabolic reactions of the alcohol functional group.

acid, UDP-glucuronate (UDPGA), to give a glucuronide (Fig. 6-4). This reaction is catalyzed by the enzyme UDP-glucuronosyltransferase (UGT). In humans the UGT proteins are produced in response to two families of genes, *UGT1* and *UGT2*, with a variety of isoforms within each of these families. The resulting glucuronide shows significant increase in water solubility normally resulting in decreased biologic activity and an increase in excretion rates. UGT is found primarily in the liver and GI tract. It should be noted that there are examples where glucuronidation increases biological activity. In the case of morphine, the morphine-6-*O*-glucuronide is 650-fold more active than morphine. In a similar fashion an alcohol can react with activated sulfuric acid, 3-phosphoadenosine-5'-phosphosulfate, to give a sulfate conjugate. This reaction is catalyzed by sulfotransferases, SULT1 or SULT2, an enzyme found in liver, intestine, kidney, and brain tissue. The sulfate conjugates also show a considerable increase in water solubility. Both the glucuronide and sulfate conjugates exhibit both hydrogen bonding and ion-dipole bonding to water accounting for the increased water solubility. For additional discussion see Appendix C, Metabolism.

Case Study 6.1

Taxanes are natural or semisynthetic macromolecules extensively used in the treatment of several cancers. They work by inhibiting cell division (mitosis) in the rapidly dividing cancer cell. While taxanes have the potential to save lives, like all anticancer agents, they are poisons and come with unwanted side effects and risks to patient welfare.

  The two taxane anticancer agents currently available in the United States are drawn below. They are both administered by the intravenous route. Since neither agent is water soluble, solubilizing agents must be added to allow the drugs to dissolve in the aqueous IV vehicle. The less water soluble agent requires Cremophor EL, which can induce a severe hypersensitivity reaction in patients. The other can get by with Tween which, while still problematic, induces less hypersensitivity than Cremophor EL. The structural segment of the two taxanes with the greatest impact on relative water solubility is circled.

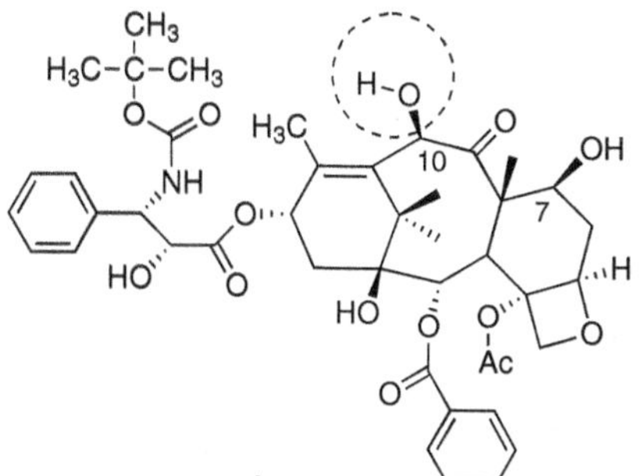

1. PV is a 59-year-old woman with metastatic breast cancer who is a candidate for taxane chemotherapy. As a younger woman she survived superficial bladder cancer, but exhibited a hypersensitivity reaction to a different drug (valrubicin) that requires Cremophor EL as a solubilizing agent. Assuming that either drug would be appropriate chemotherapy, and remembering that the less water soluble molecule would require the more problematic aqueous Cremophor EL vehicle, identify the taxane that would put PV at lower risk for another potentially serious hypersensitivity reaction. Explain your choice based on the anticipated impact of the two circled taxane moieties on water solubility.

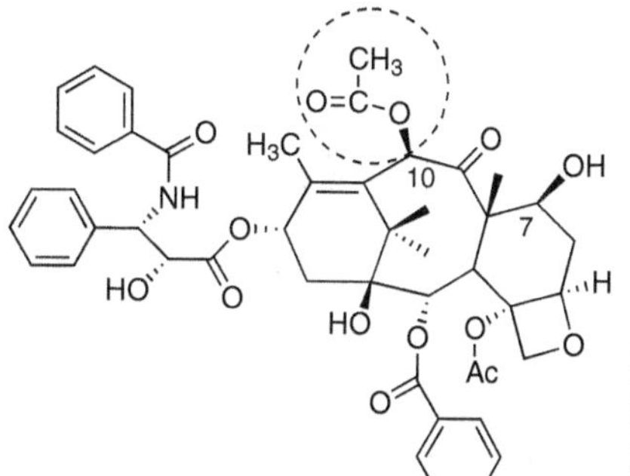

2. Note that both taxanes have a secondary alcohol at position 7. Name two potential metabolic reactions that could occur with this functional group, and then propose a reason why the taxanes are excreted with this alcohol intact (e.g., no metabolism takes place here in vivo).

Case Study 6.2

Your classmate comes to you and says that a friend sold him some capsules to help him "be smarter" on examinations. Since they have no markings, you bring them to your medicinal chemistry teacher for analysis and her preliminary evaluation is that they could be one of three phenylethylamine analogs.
Phenylethylamine is the basic pharmacophore for the neurotransmitters in the peripheral and central adrenergic (sympathetic) system. Since you are taking the organic functional group course with this professor, she uses this as a teachable moment for the class to learn about hydroxyl groups in drug molecules. You are asked to answer the following questions:

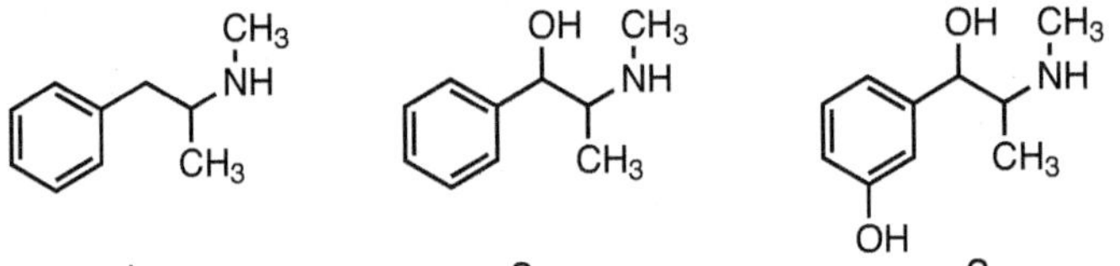

1. What functional groups, from the first six chapters of this book, are present in these phenylethylamine analogs?
2. What is the role of the hydroxyl groups in the given structures in relation to solubility in water?
3. Do each of these compounds distribute to all tissues of the body?
4. Focusing only on the aliphatic hydroxyl group in structures 2 and 3, what is its possible in vitro instability and in vivo metabolism?
5. Compound 3 was identified as the chemical in the capsules. Is your friend in trouble with the law?

Phenols

■ **NOMENCLATURE.** Phenols may appear to have some similarity to the alcohol functional group, but they are considerably different in several aspects. Phenols differ from alcohols by having the OH group attached directly to an aromatic ring. The nomenclature of the phenols is not as systematic as has been the case with the previous functional groups. In many cases, phenols are named as substituted phenols using the common ortho, meta, or para nomenclature for the location of the substituents, or the official nomenclature, in which the ring is numbered, with the carbon that bears the OH being assigned the 1 position (Fig. 7-1). In phenol nomenclature, common names are often used, such as cresol, catechol, and resorcinol. Therefore, one must be aware of these common names as well as the official nomenclature.

■ **PHYSICAL-CHEMICAL PROPERTIES.** In considering the physical properties of the phenols, one is again aware of the OH group, in which a strong electronegative group, oxygen, is attached to the electropositive hydrogen. The permanent

Structure	Common name	IUPAC name
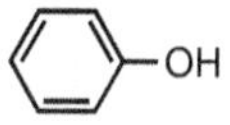 ⬡—OH	Carbolic acid	Phenol
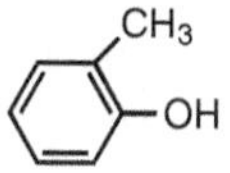 ⬡(CH₃)—OH	o-Cresol	2-Methylphenol
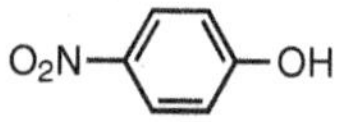 O₂N—⬡—OH	p-Nitrophenol	4-Nitrophenol
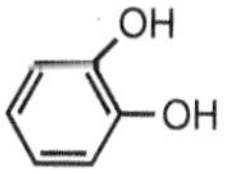 ⬡(OH)—OH	Catechol	1,2-Dihydroxybenzene
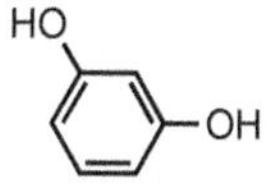 HO—⬡—OH	Resorcinol	1,3-Dihydroxybenzene
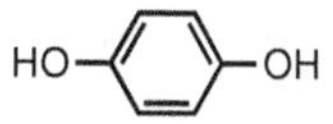 HO—⬡—OH	Hydroquinone	1,4-Dihydroxybenzene

FIGURE 7-1. Phenol nomenclature.

Table 7-1. BOILING POINTS AND WATER SOLUBILITY OF COMMON PHENOLS

	BOILING POINT °C	SOLUBILITY (g/100g H_2O)
Cyclohexanol	161	3.6
Phenol	182	9.3
p-Cresol	202	2.3
m-Chlorophenol	214	2.6
Catechol	246	45.0

dipole is capable of intermolecular hydrogen bonding, which results in high boiling points and water solubility. Added to the list of compounds in Table 7-1 is cyclohexanol. Cyclohexanol differs from phenol only in the lack of the aromatic ring. The change in the boiling point and solubility in going from cyclohexanol to phenol may seem rather large, and indeed it should be, since one property becomes important with phenols that is absent in alcohols: that property is *acidity*.

Before discussing the acidity of the phenols, let us look at some additional factors that affect solubility. As the lipophilic nature of the phenol is increased, the water solubility is decreased. The addition of a methyl (cresol) or a halogen (chlorophenol) greatly reduces the water solubility of these compounds (see Table 7-1). The addition of a second hydroxyl, such as in catechol, increases water solubility, as was the case with the previous diols. The solubility of catechol will again greatly decrease as alkyls are added to this molecule.

The acidity of phenol and substituted phenols is considered in the following illustration (Fig. 7-2). First, an acid must be defined. The classic definition states that an acid is a chemical that has the ability to give up a proton. Phenol has this ability and can therefore be considered an acid. The ease with which this proton is given up (dissociation) will influence the ratio of K_1 to K_{-1} (see Fig. 7-2). If K_1 is much greater than K_{-1}, a strong acid exists, while if K_1 is smaller than K_{-1}, a weak acid results. The factor that influences the ratio of K_1 to K_{-1} is the stability of the anion formed (in this case the phenolate anion). It should be recalled that the phenolate anion can be stabilized by resonance (i.e., the overlap of the pair of electrons on the oxygen with the delocalized cloud of electrons above and below the aromatic ring; see Fig. 7-2). This is something an alcohol cannot do because an alcohol hydroxyl is not adjacent to an aromatic system, and resonance stabilization does not occur. Therefore, dissociation of the hydrogen from the oxygen is not possible in alcohols and, by definition, the inability to give up a proton means that the alcohol is not acidic but neutral.

Let us return now to the question of boiling points and solubilities of alcohols versus phenols. Alcohols as neutral polar groups are only capable of participating

Acid (definition): $HX + H_2O \underset{K_{-1}}{\overset{K_1}{\rightleftharpoons}} H_3O^{\oplus} + X^{\ominus}$

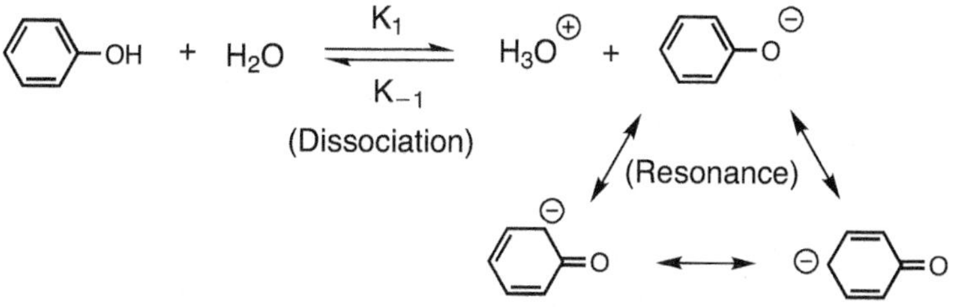

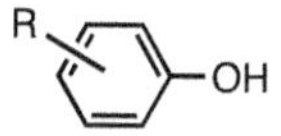

(Dissociation)

(Resonance)

R—OH	Dissociation constant	
	Ka (in water)	pKa
R = H	1.1×10^{-10}	9.96
R = m-CH$_3$	9.8×10^{-11}	10.01
R = p-CH$_3$	6.7×10^{-11}	10.17
R = m-NO$_2$	5.0×10^{-9}	8.3
R = p-NO$_2$	6.9×10^{-8}	7.16
Mineral acids	10^{-1}	1.0
Carboxylic acids	10^{-5}	5.0
Alcohols	10^{-17}	17.0

FIGURE 7-2. Dissociation constants and pKa's in water for common phenols.

in a hydrogen-bonding interaction with water. On the other hand, phenols, due to their acidity, exist both as neutral molecules and (to some extent) as ions; therefore, not only will hydrogen bonding occur, but also the stronger ion-dipole bonding can occur between the phenol and water. The prediction of a higher boiling point and a greater water solubility relates to the presence of ion-dipole interaction as well as dipole-dipole bonding.

The acidity of phenols is influenced by the substitution on the aromatic ring. Substitution ortho to the phenol affects acidity in an unpredictable manner, while substitution meta or para to the phenol results in acidities that are predictable. Substitution with a group capable of donating electrons into the aromatic ring decreases acidity. The most pronounced effect occurs when the substitution is para or in direct conjugation. Addition of an electron-withdrawing group to the aromatic ring results in increased acidity. Again, the most pronounced effect occurs with para substitution. In both cases, the influence of substituents on acidity comes from the inability or ability of the substituent to stabilize the phenolate form. Comparison of the acidity of phenols to that of carboxylic acids and mineral acids demonstrates that phenols are weak acids (Table B-1, Appendix B).

Another significant property of phenols is their chemical reactivity. An important reaction is shown in Figure 7-3. Because phenol is a weak acid, it will not react with sodium bicarbonate, a weak base, but will react with strong bases such as sodium hydroxide or potassium hydroxide to give the respective phenolate salts.

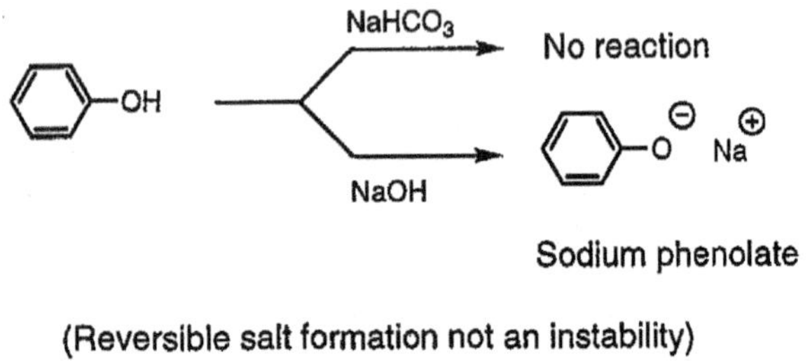

(Reversible salt formation not an instability)

FIGURE 7-3. Acid-base reaction between phenol and a strong base.

Salt formation is an important reaction since the phenolates formed are ions and will dissolve in water through the much stronger ion-dipole bonding. As salts, the simple phenols (phenol, cresol, and chlorophenol) are extremely soluble in water. Several words of caution are necessary before leaving this topic. Sodium and potassium salts will greatly increase the water solubility of the phenols. Heavy metal salts of the phenols will actually become less water-soluble because of the inability of the salt to dissociate in water. Salts of phenols that are capable of dissociation in water will always increase water solubility, and for most of the phenols of medicinal value, the salts will give enough solubility so that the drug will dissolve in water at the concentration needed for biologic activity. As the lipophilic portions attached to the aromatic ring increase, however, the solubility of the phenolate salts will decrease. *You should realize that while salt formation* (with a dissociating salt) *is an example of a chemical reaction, it is not a chemical instability.* Treatment of the water-soluble salt with acid will reverse this reaction, regenerating the phenol. For our purposes, salt formation resulting in precipitation of the organic molecule is a pharmaceutical incompatibility that the student should watch for.

A second significant chemical reaction of phenols involves their facile air oxidation. Phenols are oxidized to quinones, which are highly colored. A clear solution of phenol allowed to stand in contact with air or light soon develops a yellow coloration owing to the formation of *p*-quinone or *o*-quinone (Fig. 7-4). This reaction occurs more readily with salts of phenols and with polyphenolic compounds. Phenols and their salts must be protected from oxygen and light by being stored in closed, amber containers or by the addition of antioxidants.

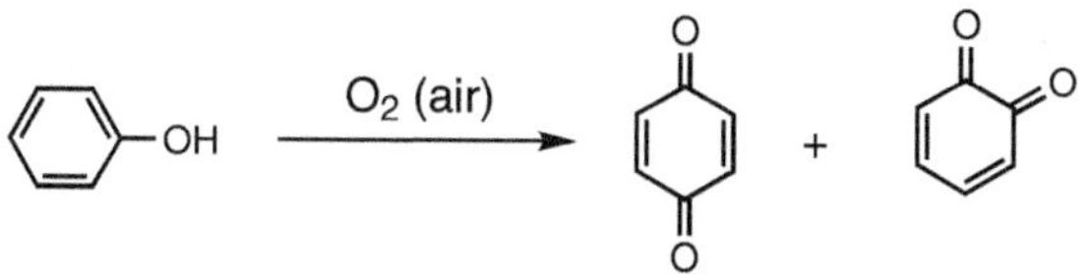

FIGURE 7-4. Oxidation of phenol with molecular oxygen.

▪ **METABOLISM.** The metabolism of phenols is much like that of alcohols. The phenol may be oxidized, or, using the terminology previously used for aromatic oxidation, the phenol may be hydroxylated, to give a diphenolic compound (Fig. 7-5) (phase 1 reaction). In most cases, the new OH group will be either ortho or para to the original hydroxyl group. Hydroxylation reactions are commonly catalyzed by members of the cytochrome P450 family of enzymes. The most common form of metabolism of phenols is conjugation with glucuronic acid to form the glucuronide or sulfonation to give the sulfate conjugate (phase 2 reaction). Both conjugation reactions give metabolites that have greater water solubility than the unmetabolized phenol. An additional type of metabolism seen to a minor extent in xenobiotics (exogenous substrates) and more common with endogenous substrates is methylation. A cofactor essential to this reaction is S-adenosylmethionine (SAM). Methylation is also considered a phase 2 reaction and the resulting methyl ether of the phenol exhibits a decreased water solubility.

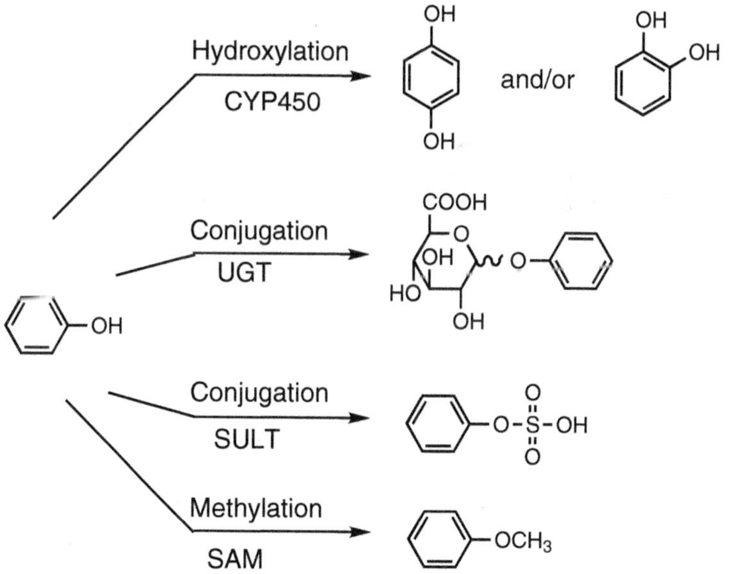

FIGURE 7-5. Metabolic reactions common to phenol functional groups.

Case Study 7.1

You are interning at "Top Flight Pharmacy" at the Strategic Air Command in Bellevue, NE. Your preceptor, Dr. I.M. Savvy, is committed to the concept that pharmacists are the chemistry experts of the health care team, and routinely encourages you to be scientifically grounded in your practice. Dr. Savvy has just discovered a bottle of "almost-expired" norepinephrine bitartrate, a cateholic adrenergic agonist used to increase blood pressure in cases of acute hypotension and to stimulate the heart in cardiac arrest. The normally clear solution has taken on a slight yellowish brown color. Dr. Savvy takes this opportunity to evaluate your understanding of in vitro drug stability by asking you to state whether this drug would be safe to use in a cardiovascular emergency, and to provide a chemical explanation for your answer.

He then asks you to predict which, if any, of the related structures drawn below might also be expected to present as a yellowish solution with time.

Finally, he asks you whether norepinephrine could/should be marketed as the sodium salt, rather than as the bitartrate salt.

How do you respond?

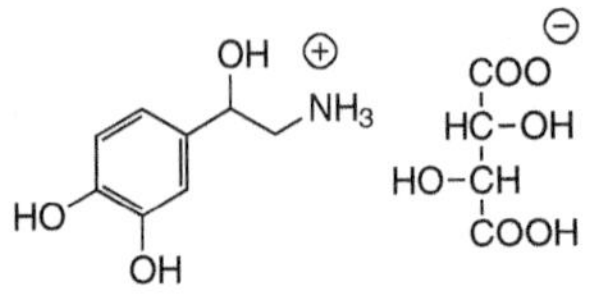

Norepinephrine bitartrate

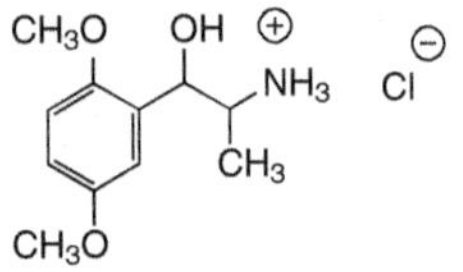

Methoxamine hydrochloride
(a vasoconstrictor)

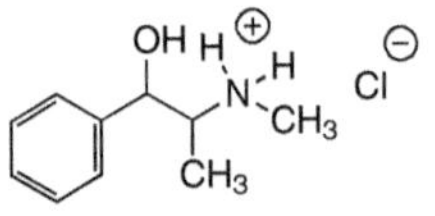

Ephedrine hydrochloride
(a vasoconstrictor)

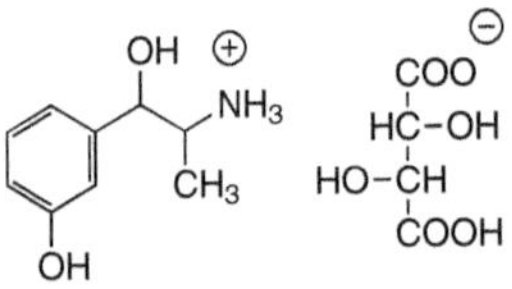

Metaraminol bitartrate
(a vasoconstrictor)

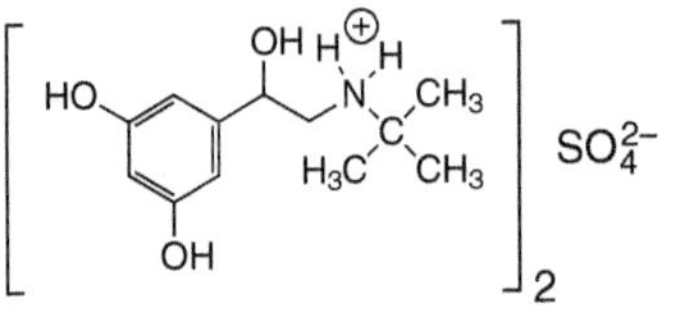

Terbutaline sulfate
(a bronchodilator)

Case Study 7.2

You are spending Spring break with your family at your summer house in South Hampton, LI. After dinner one evening you are relaxing on the porch, reading a novel and your mom comes and asks you a question. She tells you that she has been prescribed Premarin for her postmenopausal symptoms and to help prevent the development of osteoporosis. She read the package insert and understands that Premarin contains conjugated estrogens. Knowing your love of chemistry she looked up the structures of the naturally occurring estrogens found in Premarin and shown below. Her question to you is, what does the term "conjugated estrogens" mean?

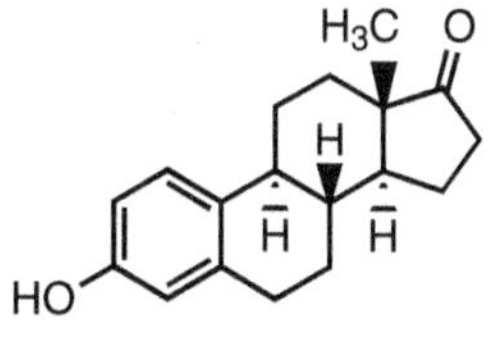

Estrone 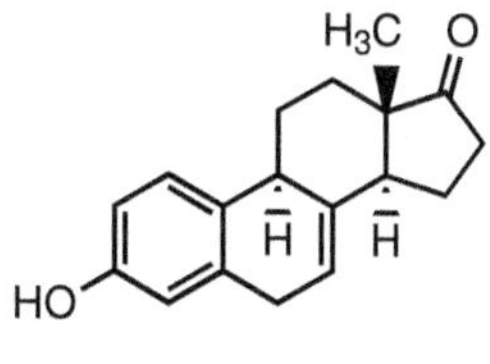   Equilin

While answering your mother's first question you say to her that these conjugated estrogens will be rapidly excreted. To which your mom then surprises you with an astute question: "Well, if the conjugated estrogens are excreted from the body how can they be available to me when I take them in the form of a pill?"

Ethers and Thioethers

ETHERS

■ **NOMENCLATURE.** Another important functional group found in many medicinal agents is the ether moiety shown in Fig. 8-1. The ethers use a common nomenclature in which the compounds are called ethers, and both substituents are named by their radical names, such as methyl, ethyl, or phenyl. Thus, Ether USP, a common name, can also be referred to as diethylether. The official names for the simple ethers are shown in Fig. 8-1. The inherent problem of naming the alkyl radical again arises as branching in the alkyl chain occurs. The official nomenclature names the compounds as alkoxy derivatives of alkanes. In the example shown below, the longest continuous alkane chain containing the ether is chosen as the base name, and the alkane is numbered to give the ether the lowest number. The correct name for the ether is therefore 2-methoxy (numbered to give the alkoxy the lowest number)-4,4-dimethylpentane (the longest alkane chain). In drug molecules the student should be able to identify the alkoxy or aryloxy groups and assign the appropriate properties.

■ **PHYSICAL-CHEMICAL PROPERTIES.** What can one predict about the water solubility of the ether group? It is interesting that the synthesis of ethers is brought about by combining two alcohols or an alcohol and phenol to give the ether. The precursors have high boiling points, strongly bond to water to give solubility, and show chemical reactivity under certain conditions. Ethers, by contrast, are low-boiling liquids with poor water solubility (Fig. 8-2) and chemically are almost inert. This becomes

Structure	Common name (Alkylalkylether)	IUPAC name
$H_3C-O-CH_2CH_3$	Ethylmethylether	Methoxyethane
$CH_3CH_2-O-CH_2CH_3$	Diethylether (Ether USP)	Ethoxyethane
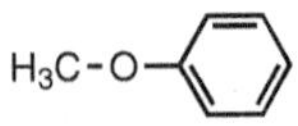 $H_3C-O-\langle\bigcirc\rangle$	Methylphenylether (Anisole)	Methoxybenzene

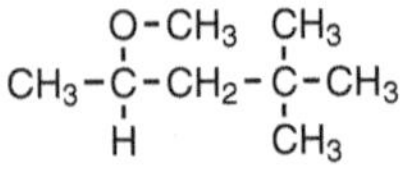

$$\begin{array}{ccccc} & O-CH_3 & CH_3 & & \\ CH_3-\underset{H}{C}-CH_2-\underset{CH_3}{C}-CH_3 & & & \\ 1 & 2 & 3 & 4 & 5 \\ 5 & 4 & 3 & 2 & 1 \end{array}$$

2-Methoxy-4,4-dimethylpentane (Correct)

4-Methoxy-2,2-dimethylpentane (Incorrect)

FIGURE 8-1. Ether nomenclature.

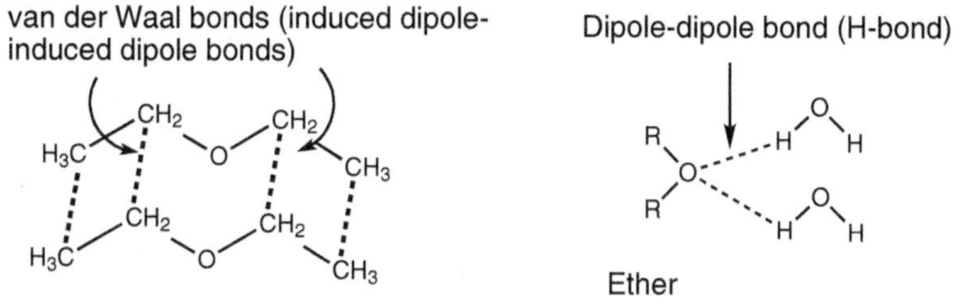

van der Waal bonds (induced dipole-induced dipole bonds)

Dipole-dipole bond (H-bond)

Ether

Ether	Boiling points (°C)	Solubility (g/100 ml H_2O)
R = C_2H_5	34.6	8.4
R = $\begin{smallmatrix}H_3C\\H_3C\end{smallmatrix}$CH−	68	0.002

FIGURE 8-2. Diagrammatic representation of the intermolecular bonding between ethers and between an ether and water accounting for low boiling points and solubility in water, respectively.

understandable when one recalls that the properties of alcohols and phenols depend primarily upon the OH group. With diethyl ether, resulting from the combination of two moles of ethanol, the OH groups have been lost. Without the OH group, hydrogen bonds cannot exist, and the only intermolecular bonding is weak van der Waals attraction and thus a low boiling point. Ether can hydrogen bond to water. The hydrogen of water will bond to the electron-rich oxygen (see Fig. 8-2). The lower-membered ethers therefore show partial water solubility, but as the hydrocarbon portion increases, water solubility rapidly decreases. In the area of general anesthetics, this water solubility for ethers has a significant effect on the onset and duration of biologic activity. The figures given for boiling points and water solubility for two ethers shown in Fig. 8-2 demonstrate the weak intermolecular bonding and how rapidly water solubility decreases as the hydrocarbon portion increases.

Chemically the ethers are relatively nonreactive, stable entities, with one important exception. Liquid ethers in contact with atmospheric oxygen form *peroxides* (Fig. 8-3). The peroxide formed, although not present in great quantities, can be quite irritating to the mucous membranes and, if concentrated, may explode. Hence, care should be taken in handling ethers to minimize the contact with oxygen. Many times an antioxidant such as copper metal is added to take up any oxygen that may be present and thus prevent this instability.

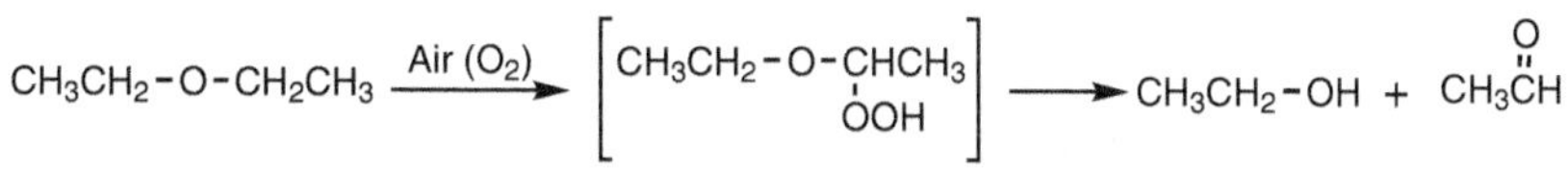

$$CH_3CH_2-O-CH_2CH_3 \xrightarrow{\text{Air } (O_2)} \left[CH_3CH_2-O-\underset{\underset{OOH}{|}}{CHCH_3} \right] \longrightarrow CH_3CH_2-OH + CH_3\overset{\overset{O}{||}}{CH}$$

FIGURE 8-3. Oxidation of an ether with molecular oxygen to give a peroxide.

■ **METABOLISM.** The metabolism of ethers in general is uneventful. With most ethers, one finds the ether excreted unchanged. There are exceptions to this rule, and the one exception that should be learned is the metabolic dealkylation reaction. When this does occur, the alkyl group that is lost is usually a small group such as a methyl or ethyl group. Metabolic dealkylation is a reaction that is catalyzed by various members of the cytochrome P450 family of enzymes. In the most common cases of dealkylation of an ether, a phenol forms, which is then metabolized by the routes of metabolism open to phenol, namely the glucuronide or sulfate conjugation. The alkyl group is lost as an aldehyde, either formaldehyde (Fig. 8-4) or acetaldehyde if the alkyl radical is ethyl.

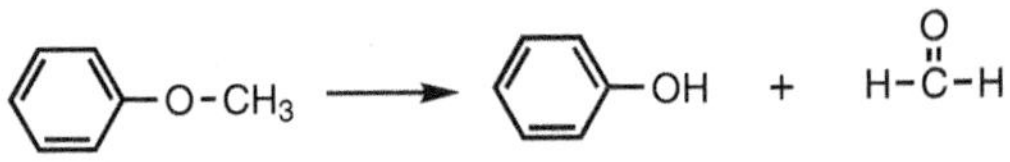

FIGURE 8-4. Metabolic dealkylation of anisole.

THIOETHERS

Nomenclature

The thioethers are also commonly referred to as the alkyl or arylthio group or alkyl or aryl mercaptans. The student is expected to identify the thioether portion of a drug molecule and associate with these groups specific physical-chemical and metabolic properties. The thioether is mentioned because it is found in a variety of drug molecules as a diaryl-, dialkyl-, or arylalkyl thioether (Fig. 8-5).

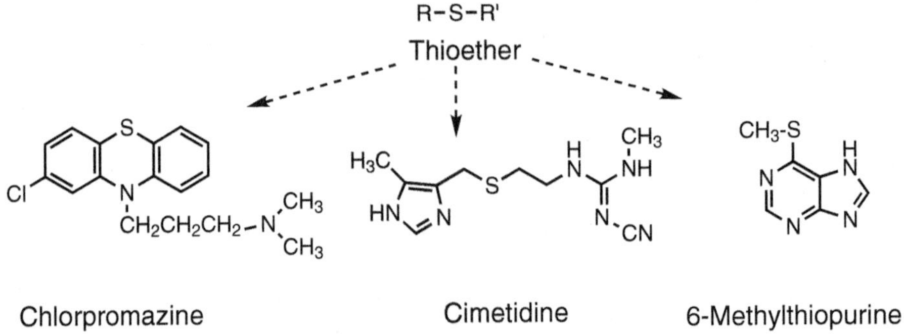

FIGURE 8-5. Examples of the thioether in drug molecules.

Physical-Chemical Properties

The replacement of oxygen with sulfur results in a compound with a significant increase in the boiling point (diethyl thioether, 92°) and a decrease in water solubility (diethyl thioether insoluble). In general, the thioether should be considered to be lipophilic functional groups.

Metabolism

Thioethers may undergo one of two metabolic reactions depending on the nature of the thio substituents. Of significance is the unique metabolic oxidation reaction that thioethers may undergo. The oxidation reaction may not be too surprising since sulfur exists in a variety of oxidation states including -2, $+4$, and $+6$. The thioether moiety may undergo a single oxidation to the sulfoxide or may be oxidized to the sulfone (Fig. 8-6). This reaction is catalyzed by flavin mono-oxygenase (FMO).

In a process similar to that experienced by short-chain alkylethers, short-chain alkyl thioethers may undergo dealkylation giving rise to a thiol and an aldehyde. This reaction is catalyzed by cytochrome family of enzymes.

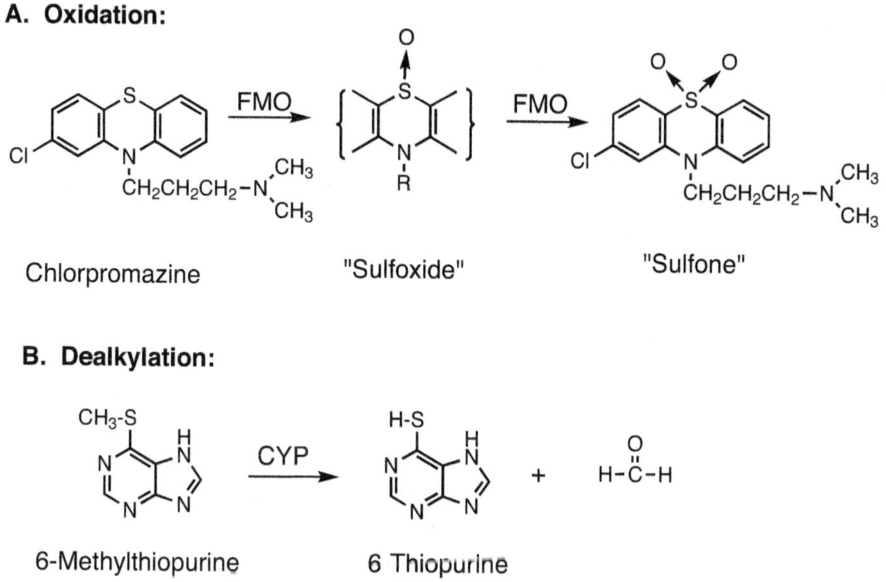

A. Oxidation:

Chlorpromazine   "Sulfoxide"   "Sulfone"

B. Dealkylation:

6-Methylthiopurine   6 Thiopurine

FIGURE 8-6. Metabolism of thioethers.

THIOL OXIDATION

While not common in drug molecules, the thiol functional group is very common in protein structures as it is present in the amino acid cysteine (see Chapter 15). A thiol functional group is readily oxidized by molecular oxygen to a disulfide dimer. An example of such an instability is seen with the

(continued)

THIOL OXIDATION (continued)

drug captopril which is oxidized in solution to its dimer. The thiol–disulfide interconversion plays a significant role in the three-dimensional structure of proteins.

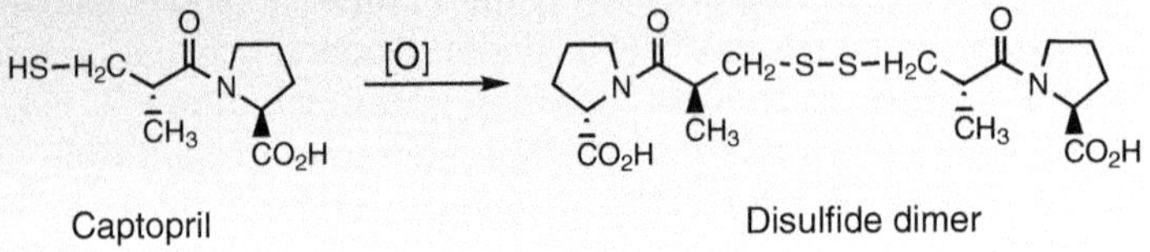

Captopril   Disulfide dimer

Case Study 8.1

Opioid analgesics are potent pain relievers that work in the brain and spinal cord (CNS). Some opioids are found in nature, including the two structures drawn below.

1. Use your understanding of organic functional group properties to predict whether opioid **1** or opioid **2** would more effectively penetrate the blood-brain barrier and concentrate at the site of action.

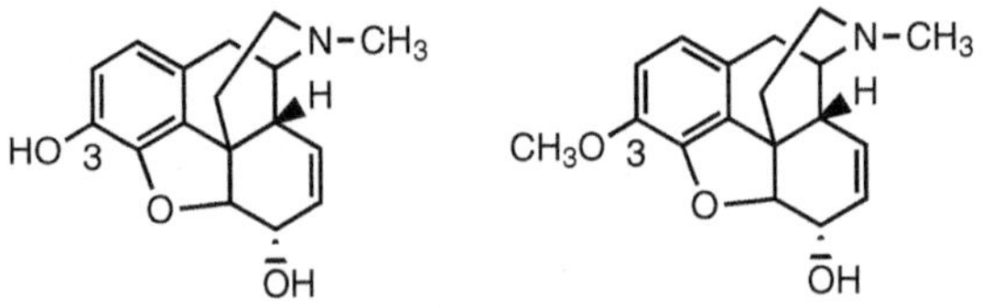

               1   **2**

2. Opioid **1** is 10 to 12 times more potent as a pain reliever than opioid **2**. Reflect on your response to the distribution question just answered, and propose an explanation for this therapeutic reality.
3. The following is based on a true story: Mrs. X is a woman of poor CYP2D6 metabolizing phenotype who gave birth to a healthy baby boy. As a result of her genetic profile (few, if any, functional CYP2D6 enzymes), she was given high doses of opioid **2** for episiotomy pain. Opioid **2** is excreted in breast milk, and Mrs. X was nursing her newborn. Within a few days of his birth, Mrs. X's son became lethargic and subsequently died of respiratory depression (a direct result of opioid overdose). Explain the chemistry behind this tragic outcome, and identify what you, as the pharmacist, could have done to prevent it.

Case Study 8.2

As part of your early practice experiences you have elected to rotate through the outpatient surgery unit at the local hospital. This week, you will be observing a traditional open-shoulder rotator cuff repair where the patient will be under general anesthesia using a volatile ether anesthetic. The key to doing this procedure on an outpatient basis is a rapid recovery from the general anesthesia. During your observation of the patient's evaluation, the anesthesiologist turns to you and says "We have the following three volatile ether anesthetics (see below), which one would you recommend for this surgery?"

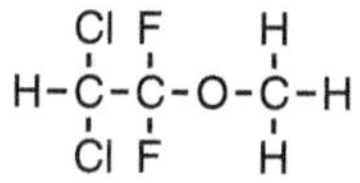

$$
\begin{array}{ccc}
\underset{\underset{Cl}{|}}{\overset{\overset{Cl}{|}}{H-C}}-\underset{\underset{F}{|}}{\overset{\overset{F}{|}}{C}}-O-\underset{\underset{H}{|}}{\overset{\overset{H}{|}}{C}}-H
&
\underset{\underset{Cl}{|}}{\overset{\overset{F}{|}}{H-C}}-\underset{\underset{F}{|}}{\overset{\overset{F}{|}}{C}}-O-\underset{\underset{F}{|}}{\overset{\overset{F}{|}}{C}}-H
&
\underset{\underset{F}{|}}{\overset{\overset{F}{|}}{F-C}}-\underset{\underset{H}{|}}{\overset{\overset{F}{|}}{C}}-O-\underset{\underset{F}{|}}{\overset{\overset{F}{|}}{C}}-H
\end{array}
$$

Methoxyflurane	Enflurane	Desflurane
oil/gas = 970	oil/gas = 98.5	oil/gas = 16.7
blood/gas = 12	blood/gas = 1.1	blood/gas = 0.42

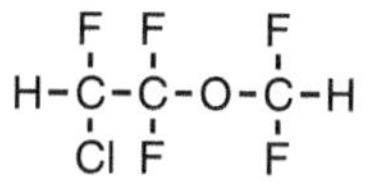

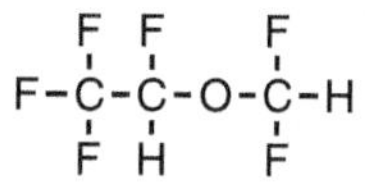

You remember when you studied ethers in the organic functional groups course that the relative water solubility has a significant effect on the onset and duration of action of the volatile ether anesthetics. The water solubility of volatile ether anesthetics is usually expressed as their blood/gas ratio and this ratio directly correlates to the oil/gas ratio that is easier to measure. The higher this ratio is, the greater the blood/gas ratio of the ether.

Aldehydes and Ketones

■ **NOMENCLATURE.** Two functional groups that, owing to their chemical and physical similarities, can be grouped together are the aldehydes and ketones. From the examples of common names shown in Figure 9-1, one can see that the structural identity of simple aldehydes and ketones is obvious since the term "aldehyde" or "ketone" appears in the nomenclature. The common nomenclature for aldehydes remains useful until one is unable to name the alkyl radical that contains the **carbonyl**, and then the formal IUPAC name is used. The longest continuous chain containing the aldehyde functional group is chosen as the base name and numbered such that the aldehyde constitutes the 1 position. To show the presence of an aldehyde in the molecule, the suffix "-al" replaces the "e" in the alkane base name. Hence, the more complex structure A shown in Figure 9-1 is named 3,3-dimethylbutanal.

With the common nomenclature of ketones, as indicated, the word "ketone" is used as part of the nomenclature. With ketones, the two radicals attached to the carbonyl are individually named until these radical names become unwieldy. The IUPAC rules for ketones require that one find the longest continuous carbon chain that contains the ketone and number so as to give the lowest number to the carbonyl group. If the ketone is at the same location from either end of the molecule, then the correct direction of numbering is the one that gives the lowest number to any remaining substituents. The designation used to show the presence of a ketone carbonyl is the suffix "-one" which, along with the ketone location, replaces the "e" in the alkane base name. The example given for structure B in Figure 9-1 becomes 2,5,7,7-tetramethyl-4-(the location of the carbonyl) octan (specifying an 8-carbon chain)-one (the abbreviation for a ketone).

It should be noted that a carbon atom attached to an oxygen atom through a double bond is defined as a carbonyl. A carbonyl is not considered an organic functional group, but is found in a variety of organic functional groups such as aldehydes, ketones, carboxylic acids, etc. With drugs that have complex IUPAC nomenclature, the student is expected to correctly identify the presence of a carbonyl and assign this group to an appropriate functional group category such as an aldehyde or ketone and may then use this generic nomenclature.

■ **PHYSICAL-CHEMICAL PROPERTIES.** In considering the properties of aldehydes and ketones, it must be noted that the carbonyl group present in both molecules is polar, and hence the compounds are polar. Oxygen is more electronegative than carbon, and the cloud of electrons that makes up the carbon-oxygen double bond is therefore distorted toward the oxygen. In addition, ketones and to a

Structure	Common name	IUPAC name
Aldehydes:		
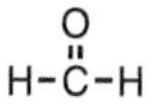 $H-\overset{\overset{O}{\parallel}}{C}-H$	Formaldehyde	Methanal
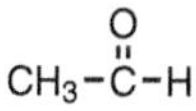 $CH_3-\overset{\overset{O}{\parallel}}{C}-H$	Acetaldehyde	Ethanal
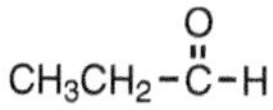 $CH_3CH_2-\overset{\overset{O}{\parallel}}{C}-H$	Propionaldehyde	Propanal
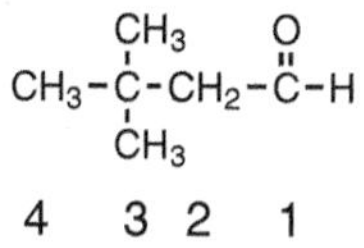 $CH_3-\overset{CH_3}{\underset{CH_3}{C}}-CH_2-\overset{\overset{O}{\parallel}}{C}-H$ 4 3 2 1	Structure A	3,3-Dimethylbutanal -al = aldehyde
Ketones:		
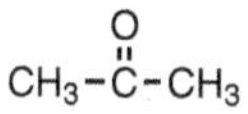 $CH_3-\overset{\overset{O}{\parallel}}{C}-CH_3$	Dimethylketone (Acetone)	2-Propanone
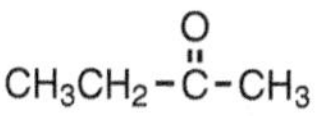 $CH_3CH_2-\overset{\overset{O}{\parallel}}{C}-CH_3$	Ethylmethylketone	2-Butanone
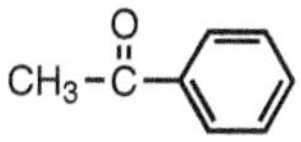 $CH_3-\overset{\overset{O}{\parallel}}{C}-\bigcirc$	Methylphenylketone (Acetophenone)	1-Phenylethanone
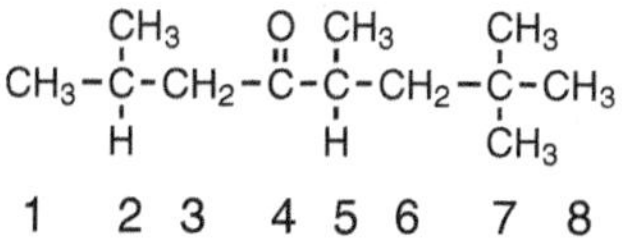 $CH_3-\underset{H}{\overset{CH_3}{C}}-CH_2-\overset{\overset{O}{\parallel}}{C}-\underset{H}{\overset{CH_3}{C}}-CH_2-\overset{CH_3}{\underset{CH_3}{C}}-CH_3$ 1 2 3 4 5 6 7 8	Structure B	2,5,7,7-Tetramethyl-4-octanone -one = ketone

FIGURE 9-1. Aldehyde and ketone nomenclature.

lesser extent aldehydes may exist in equilibrium with the "enol" form (Fig. 9-2). This property and the polar nature of the carbonyl lead to higher boiling points for aldehydes and ketones compared with nonpolar compounds of comparable molecular weight. Because of the high electron density on the oxygen atom, aldehydes and ketones can hydrogen bond to water and will dissolve, to some extent, in water. The hydrogen bonding is similar to that suggested for ethers but stronger. Keep in mind that as the nonpolar hydrocarbon portion increases, the

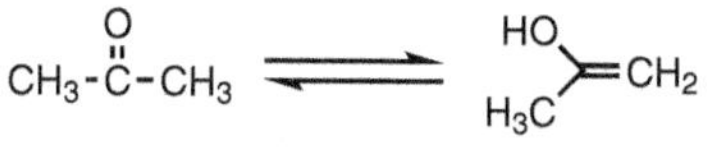

$$CH_3-\overset{\overset{O}{\parallel}}{C}-CH_3 \rightleftharpoons \underset{H_3C}{\overset{HO}{>}}=CH_2$$

"Keto"   "Enol"

FIGURE 9-2. "Keto" – "enol" equilibrium of acetone.

Table 9-1. BOILING POINTS AND WATER SOLUBILITY OF COMMON ALDEHYDES AND KETONES

$R-\overset{\overset{\text{O}}{\|}}{C}-H$			$R-\overset{\overset{\text{O}}{\|}}{C}-R'$			
	BOILING POINT	SOLUBILITY			BOILING POINT	SOLUBILITY
R	°C	(g/100g H_2O)	R	R'	°C	(g/100g H_2O)
H	−21	∞	CH_3	CH_3	56	∞
CH_3	20	∞	CH_3	C_2H_5	80	26.0
C_2H_5	49	16.0	CH_3	$n\text{-}C_3H_7$	102	6.3
$n\text{-}C_3H_7$	76	7.0	C_2H_5	C_2H_5	101	5.0
C_6H_5	178	0.3	C_6H_5	CH_3	202	<1.0

effect of the polar carbonyl group on overall solubility will decrease. This is illustrated in Table 9-1, where it is apparent that as the hydrocarbon portion increases beyond two or three carbons, the water solubility decreases rapidly in both aldehydes and ketones. Some water solubility is still possible, however, with a total carbon content of five or six carbons.

In considering the chemical reactivity from a pharmaceutical standpoint, the ketone functional group is relatively nonreactive. This is not true of the aldehyde functional group. Aldehydes are one oxidation state from the stable carboxylic acid structure, and most are therefore rapidly oxidized. With many liquids, this means air oxidation, and compounds containing aldehydes therefore must be protected from atmospheric oxygen. The low-molecular-weight aldehydes can also undergo polymerization to cyclic trimers, a compound containing three aldehyde units, or straight-chain polymers (Fig. 9-3). The trimers are stable to oxygen but will allow regeneration of the aldehyde upon heating. In some cases, this reaction is used advantageously to protect the aldehyde.

A sequence of chemical reactions common to both aldehydes and ketones is the reaction that occurs between aldehydes or ketones and alcohols (Fig. 9-4). This

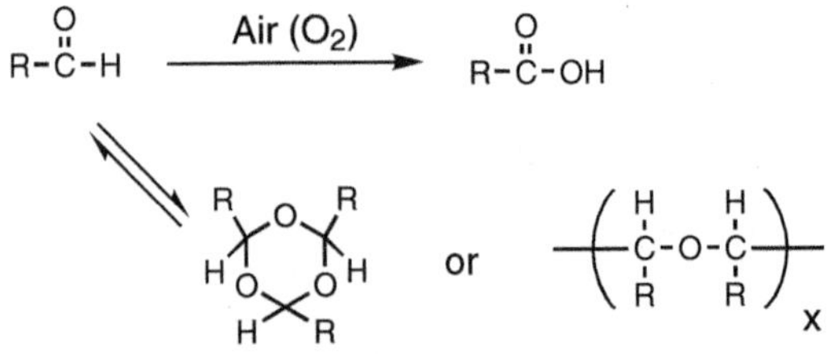

FIGURE 9-3. Oxidation and polymerization reactions of aldehydes.

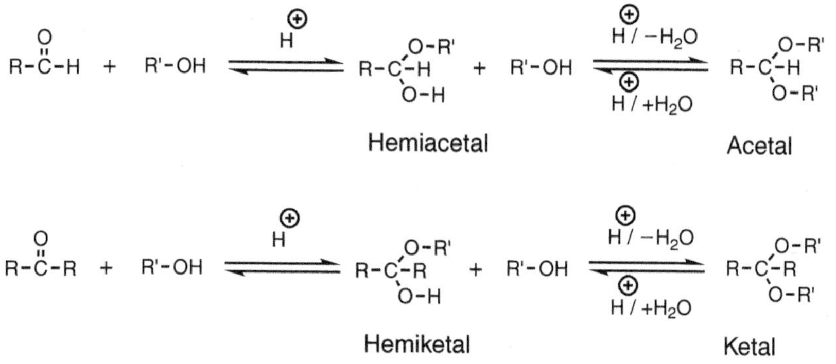

FIGURE 9-4. Formation of acetals and ketals from aldehydes and ketones, respectively.

reaction is catalyzed by acid. The reaction leading to hemiacetals or hemiketals and acetals or ketals is significant in that some drugs and many drug metabolites exist as one of these derivatives. The reaction of an aldehyde with an alcohol under acidic conditions gives a hemiacetal. "Hemi" refers to half, in this case half an acetal. The hemiacetal is unstable to aqueous conditions, irrespective of pH. Further addition of a second alcohol to the hemiacetal can occur, leading to an acetal. Acetals are stable to aqueous conditions at neutral or basic pH but are unstable to aqueous acidic conditions, with conversion back to the aldehyde occurring. In a similar manner, a ketone may be converted to a hemiketal and further to a ketal by reaction with an alcohol under acidic conditions. The same stability properties exist for hemiketals and ketals as was mentioned for acetals. Probably the best examples of acetals are the glucuronides formed between alcohols or phenols with glucuronic acid, while an example of an hemiacetal is the sugar glucuronic acid itself. In these cases the hemiacetal is an intramolecular hemiacetal (Fig. 9-5). The aminoglycoside antibiotics represent a drug class that possesses the acetal functional group, and the previously mentioned polymers of aldehydes are also examples of acetals.

▪ **METABOLISM.** Several possible metabolic routes are found in vivo for aldehydes and ketones. Aldehydes in general are readily oxidized by xanthine oxidase, aldehyde oxidase, and NAD-specific aldehyde dehydrogenase, the resulting product being a carboxylic acid (Fig. 9-6). These oxidative enzymes are not cytochrome P450-associated enzymes.

Ketones are fairly stable in vivo toward oxidation, although with an aromatic alkyl ketone, an oxidation reaction may occur to give an aromatic acid (Fig. 9-7).

A second metabolic reaction that may affect aldehydes and ketones is reduction. While reduction appears to be a minor metabolic reaction for aldehydes (Fig. 9-7), many ketones, especially α, β-unsaturated ketones, undergo reduction to a secondary alcohol. This reaction is often **stereoselective**, giving rise primarily to one isomer (Fig. 9-8).

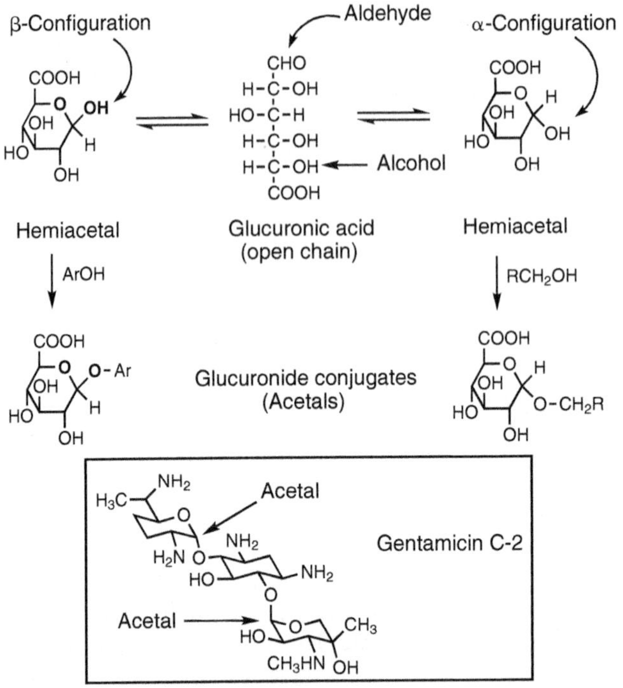

FIGURE 9-5. Glucuronic acid as an aldehyde and hemiacetal.

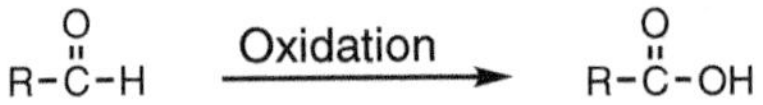

Oxidizing enzymes: Xanthine oxidase
Aldehyde oxidase
Aldehyde dehydrogenase

FIGURE 9-6. Metabolic oxidation of aldehydes.

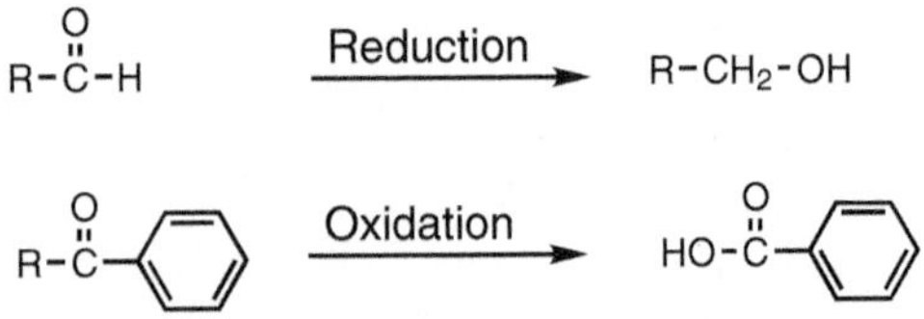

FIGURE 9-7. Minor metabolic reactions of aldehydes and ketones.

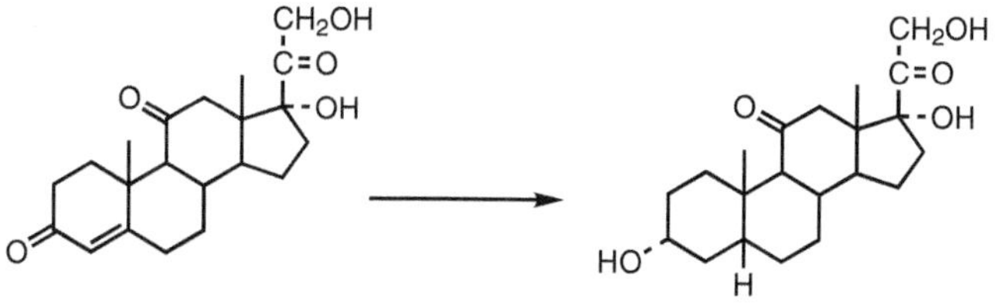

FIGURE 9-8. Metabolism of cortisone to tetrahydrocortisone.

Case Study 9.1

As a socially conscious health care practitioner, you consult with a drug abuse re-habilitation clinic and analytical laboratory in your community. An analytical chemist has just phoned you about PT, a 28-year-old heroin addict who was ad-mitted a month ago to a supervised methadone maintenance program. This re-covering patient has been receiving methadone on schedule. Yesterday he presented for a "spot check" urinalysis as requested by his employer.

The chemist has identified a compound in PT's urine that has him worried. Concerned that PT might be engaged in illicit drug-seeking behavior, he wants to know if this strange compound could possibly be related to PT's legitimate methadone administration, or whether he should notify the clinic director and PT's probation officer about his suspicions.

In preparing to answer this chemist's question, you remind yourself of three important chemical realities:

1. Methadone undergoes CYP-mediated N-dealkylation in vivo to provide the pri-mary amine dinormethadone
2. Amines (like alcohols) have a nucleophilic lone pair of electrons
3. Tertiary alcohols dehydrate to generate olefins (carbon-carbon double bonds)

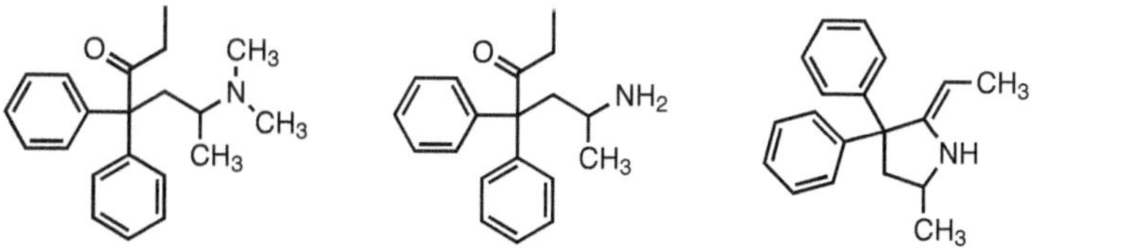

| Methadone | Dinormethadone | Compound identified in PT's urine |

So what do you think? Is PT condemned or exonerated by his own urine sample?

Case Study 9.2

Dr. V, a dermatologist, has sought your advice in regard to compounding an oleaginous ointment containing a corticosteroid for the treatment of his patient's psoriasis. He wants the steroid's duration of action to be prolonged, which requires that the drug be highly soluble in the ointment so that its release from the vehicle is slow. Dr. V says that since you are a compounding pharmacist, he is confident that you will be able to make the special lipophilic ointment formulation (see Dr. V's prescription) that he wants to use to incorporate the steroid. However, he is not sure which of the three triamcinolone-based compounds, shown below, would provide the longest duration of action in this compounded product, and asks your opinion. Analyze the three structures and make a recommendation.

Dr. V's Rx for 0.05% Corticosteroid Ointment:

Corticosteroid	0.50 mg/g
Propylene glycol monostearate	120.00 mg/g
White wax USP	60.00 mg/g
White petrolatum	819.50 mg/g

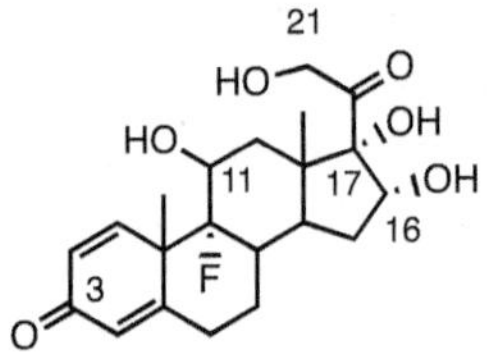

Triamcinolone 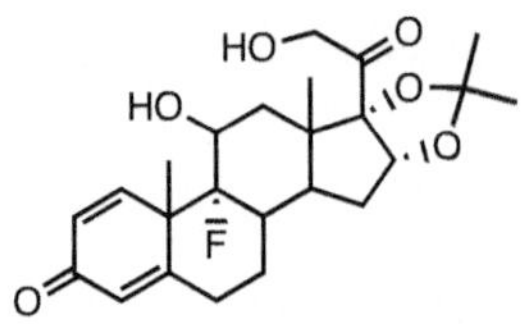   Triamcinolone acetonide 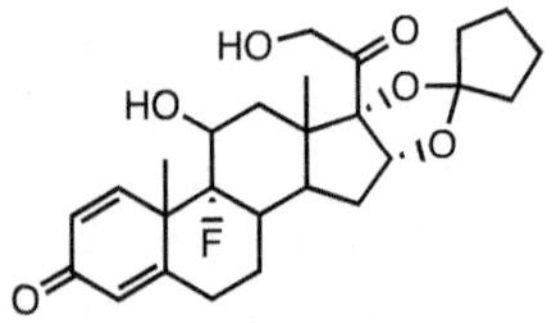   Triamcinolone cyclopentonide

Amines

AMINES—GENERAL

Two major functional groups still remain to be considered. These two groups, the carboxylic acids and the amines, are extremely important to medicinal chemistry and especially to the solubility nature of organic medicinals. In addition, the functional derivatives of these groups will be considered. In many instances the carboxylic acid or amine functional group is added to organic molecules with the specific purpose of promoting water solubility, since it is generally found that compounds showing little or no water solubility also are devoid of biologic activity.

■ **NOMENCLATURE.** The common nomenclature for amines is illustrated in Figure 10-1. Inspection of this nomenclature reveals that the common names consist of the name of the alkyl or aryl radical, followed by the word "amine." The examples given also show the different types of amines. The primary amine, isopropylamine, has a single substituent attached to the nitrogen; the secondary amine, ethylmethylamine, has two substituents attached to the nitrogen. The tertiary amine, *t*-butylethylmethylamine, has three groups attached directly to the

Structure	Common name (Alkylamine)	IUPAC name
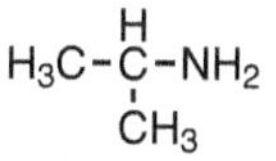 $H_3C-\overset{H}{\underset{CH_3}{C}}-NH_2$	Isopropylamine (Primary amine)	2-Aminopropane
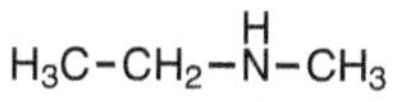 $H_3C-CH_2-\overset{H}{N}-CH_3$	Ethylmethylamine (Secondary amine)	N-Methylaminoethane
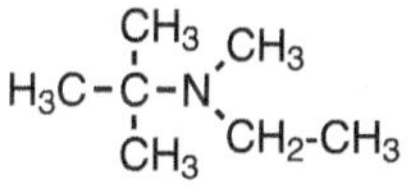 $H_3C-\overset{CH_3}{\underset{CH_3}{C}}-N\overset{CH_3}{\underset{CH_2-CH_3}{}}$	*t*-Butylethylmethylamine (Tertiary amine)	N-Ethyl-N-methyl-2-methyl-2-aminopropane
$\begin{array}{c}C_6H_5 \quad CH_3\\ \quad N-\overset{}{\underset{H}{C}}-CH_2-CH_2-CH_3\\ H_3C-CH\\ \quad CH_3\end{array}$	N-Phenyl-N-(2-propyl)-2-aminopentane N = substituent on the Nitrogen	

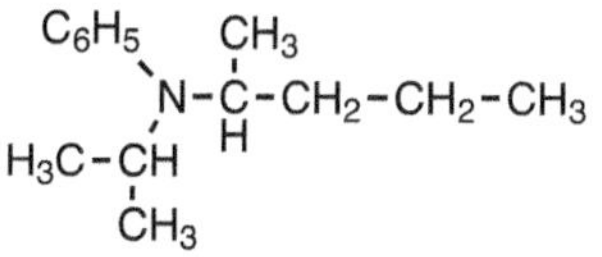

FIGURE 10-1. Amine nomenclature.

nitrogen. As with all common nomenclatures, the system becomes nearly impossible to use as the branching of the alkyl groups increases, and the official nomenclature becomes necessary. In the IUPAC system, the amines are considered substituted alkanes. The longest continuous alkyl chain containing the amine is identified and serves as the base name. The alkane chain is numbered in such a manner as to give the lowest possible number to the amine functional group, while the other substituents on the amine group are designated by use of a capital "N" before the name of the substituents. Examples are given in Figure 10-1.

■ **PHYSICAL-CHEMICAL PROPERTIES.** The amine functional group is probably one of the most common functional groups found in medicinal agents, and its value in the drug is twofold. One role is in solubilizing the drug either as the free base or as a water-soluble salt of the amine. The second role of the amine is to act as a binding site that holds the drug to a specific site in the body to produce the biologic activity. This latter role is beyond the scope of this book, but the former role contributes to an important physical property of the amine. First, let us pose a question: What influence will the amine functional group have on solubility properties? While amines are polar compounds, they may not show high boiling points or good water solubility. One reason for this is that in the tertiary amine, one does not find an electropositive group attached to the nitrogen. In the primary and secondary amines, one does have an electropositive hydrogen connected to the nitrogen, but the nitrogen is not as electronegative as oxygen, and the dipole is therefore weak. What all this means is that the amount of the intermolecular hydrogen bonding is minimal in primary and secondary amines and nonexistent in tertiary amines. This leads to relatively low-boiling liquids.

In considering water solubility, a different factor must be taken into account. The amine has an unshared pair of electrons, which leads to high electron density around the nitrogen. This high electron density promotes water solubility because hydrogen bonding between the hydrogen of water and the electron-dense nitrogen occurs. This is similar to the situation with low-molecular-weight ethers but occurs to a greater extent with basic amines. Both boiling points and the solubility effects are shown in Table 10-1. Also illustrated in Table 10-1 is the effect on solubility of increasing the hydrocarbon constituent. Primary amines tend to be more soluble than secondary amines, which are more soluble than tertiary amines. The amine can solubilize up to six or seven methylenes, which, from a solubility standpoint, makes the amines equivalent to an alcohol.

An extremely important property of the amines is their basicity and ability to form salts. The Brønsted definition of a base is the ability of a compound to accept a proton from an acid. Amines have an unshared pair of electrons, which is more or less available for sharing. The statement "more or less" has to do with the strength of a base, and this is considered in Figure 10-2. The strength of a base is defined by its relative ability to donate its unshared pair of electrons. The more readily the electrons are donated, the stronger the base. To define the strength of a base and to place this value on the same scale with acids, the measure of basicity of an amine is obtained by considering the acidity of the conjugate acid produced by protonating the amine. This protonation gives an ammonium ion and its

Table 10-1. BOILING POINTS AND WATER SOLUBILITY OF COMMON AMINES

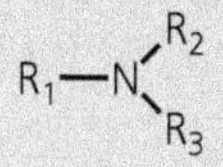

$$R_1 - N \begin{smallmatrix} R_2 \\ \\ R_3 \end{smallmatrix}$$

R_1	R_2	R_3	BOILING POINT °C	SOLUBILITY (g/100g H_2O)
CH_3	H	H	−7.5	very soluble
CH_3	CH_3	H	7.5	very soluble
CH_3	CH_3	CH_3	3.0	91.0
C_2H_5	H	H	17.0	miscible
C_2H_5	C_2H_5	H	55.0	very soluble
C_2H_5	C_2H_5	C_2H_5	89.0	14.0
C_6H_5	H	H	184.0	3.7
C_6H_5	CH_3	H	196.0	slightly soluble
C_6H_5	CH_3	CH_3	194.0	1.4

dissociation constant is given as its pK_a. Therefore, a strong base is a substance that prefers to hold on to the proton, exist as the ammonium ion, and possess a small dissociation constant (K_a) and thus a large pK_a (Example 1). On the other hand, a weak base is a substance that does not readily donate its electrons and forms an unstable ammonium ion that dissociates readily with a large dissociation constant (K_a), and thus has a small pK_a (Example 2). Another way to view this relationship is that $pK_a = 14 - pK_b$. This may be of value since older references may define bases in terms of their K_b dissociation constant and the pK_b of a base.

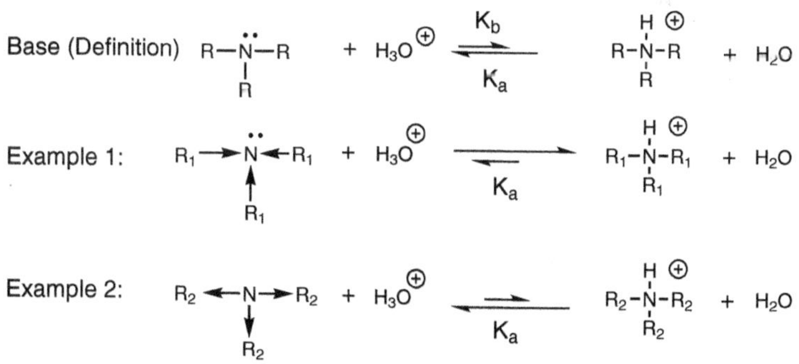

FIGURE 10-2. The influence of electron-releasing and electron-withdrawing groups on the basicity of amines.

Two factors influence basicity through the effects these factors have on the availability of the electrons. One of the factors is electronic, while the other is steric. To consider the former, if electron-donating groups are attached to the basic nitrogen, electrons are pushed into the nitrogen. Since a negative repels a negative, the electron pair on the nitrogen will be pushed out from the nitrogen, thus making the pair more readily available for donating.

If, on the other hand, electron-withdrawing or electron-attracting groups are attached to the nitrogen, the unshared pair of electrons will be pulled to the nitrogen atom and will be less readily available for donating, and therefore a weaker base results. An example of the electron donor is the alkyl, and an example of an electron-withdrawing group is the aryl or phenyl group. Based on this, one would predict that secondary alkyl amines with two electron-releasing groups attached to the nitrogen should be more basic than primary alkyl amines with a single alkyl group attached to the nitrogen. This is normally true. One would also predict that tertiary alkyl amines with three electron-releasing groups attached to the nitrogen should be more basic than secondary amines. This would be true if it were not for steric hindrance, the second factor that affects basicity. If large alkyl groups surround the unshared pair of electrons, then the approach of hydronium ions, a source of a proton, is hindered. The degree of this hindrance will affect the strength of basicity. The steric effect becomes important for tertiary amines but has little if any effect on primary and secondary amines. As shown in Figure 10-3, with amines, the large alkyl groups move back and forth, blocking the approach of water. Salt formation therefore does not occur as readily as it would in the absence

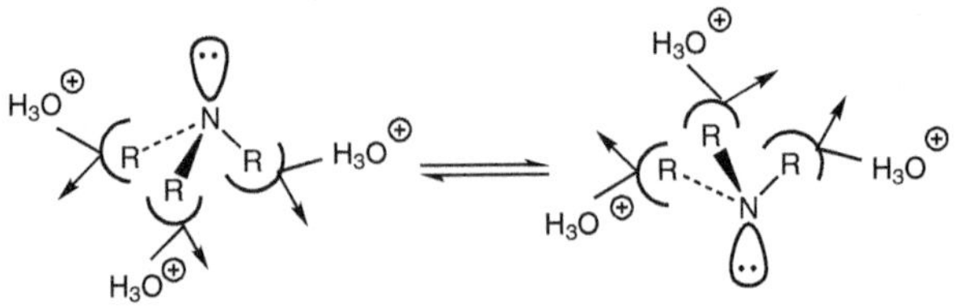

FIGURE 10-3. Diagrammatic representation of the influence of steric factors on the basicity of tertiary alkyl amines.

of such hindrance. We commonly find that with alkyl amines, secondary amines are more basic than tertiary amines, and tertiary amines are more basic than primary amines.

Aromatic amines differ significantly from alkyl amines in basicity. The aromatic ring, with its delocalized cloud of electrons, serves as an electron sink. The aromatic ring thus acts as an electron-withdrawing group, leading to a drop in basicity by six powers of ten (much lower pK_a). The unshared pair of electrons is said to be resonance stabilized, as shown in Figure 10-4. The spreading of the electron density over a greater area decreases the ability of the molecule to donate the electrons, and basicity is therefore reduced. Additional substitution on the nitrogen of

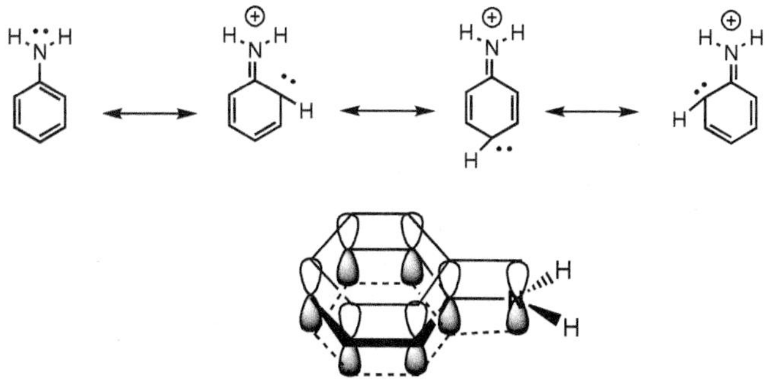

FIGURE 10-4. Resonance stabilization of an amine's unshared electron pair.

aniline with an alkyl or a second aryl group changes the basicity in a predictable manner, with the alkyl group increasing basicity and an aryl reducing basicity to a nearly neutral compound (Table 10-2). Finally, substitution on the aromatic ring also affects basicity. Substitution meta or para to the amine has a predictable effect on basicity, while ortho substitution affects basicity in an unpredictable manner (see Table 10-2). An electron-withdrawing group attached to the aromatic ring in the meta or para position decreases basicity. The decrease is significant if this group is para rather than meta. Electron-donating groups in the meta or para position usually increase basicity above that of aniline (a higher pK_a). The increase in basicity is most pronounced if the group is in the para position and not as pronounced if it is in the meta position. It should be noted that this is the same effect seen with phenols, but moving in the opposite direction. An electron-donating group attached meta or para to a phenol increases the pK_a of a phenol resulting in a less acidic or more basic phenol. With ortho-substituted anilines, predictability fails because of intramolecular interactions.

Since amines are basic, one would expect that they react with acids to form salts. This is an important reaction, for if the salts that are formed dissociate in water, there is a strong likelihood that these salts will be water-soluble (Fig. 10-5). Such is the case with many organic drugs. If a basic amine is present in the drug, it can be converted into a salt, which in turn is used to prepare aqueous solutions of the drug. The most frequently used acids for preparing salts are hydrochloric, sulfuric,

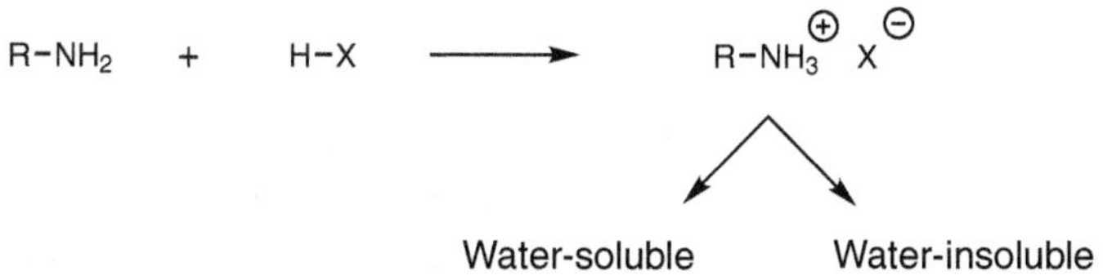

FIGURE 10-5. The salt formed from an amine and an acid is water-soluble if the salt is able to dissociate and is water-insoluble if the salt is unable to dissociate.

Table 10-2. pKa VALUES IN WATER OF COMMON PROTONATED AMINES

$$R_1-\overset{\overset{R_2}{|}\oplus}{\underset{\underset{R_3}{|}}{N}}-H \;+\; H_2O \quad\overset{K_a}{\underset{\longleftarrow}{\longrightarrow}}\quad R_1-N\overset{R_2}{\underset{R_3}{\diagup}} \;+\; H_3O^{\oplus}$$

R_1	R_2	R_3	pK_a
CH_3	H	H	10.62
CH_3CH_2	H	H	10.64
$(CH_3)_3C$	H	H	10.68
$CH_3(CH_2)_2$	H	H	10.58
CH_3	CH_3	H	10.71
CH_3CH_2	CH_3CH_2	H	10.92
$CH_3(CH_2)_2$	$CH_3(CH_2)_2$	H	10.91
CH_3	CH_3	CH_3	9.78
CH_3CH_2	CH_3CH_2	CH_3CH_2	10.75
C_6H_5	H	H	4.62
C_6H_5	CH_3	H	4.85
$p\text{-}O_2N\text{-}C_6H_4$	H	H	1.00
$m\text{-}O_2N\text{-}C_6H_4$	H	H	2.51
$p\text{-}Cl\text{-}C_6H_4$	H	H	3.98
$m\text{-}Cl\text{-}C_6H_4$	H	H	3.52
$p\text{-}CH_3\text{-}C_6H_4$	H	H	5.08
$m\text{-}CH_3\text{-}C_6H_4$	H	H	4.69
$p\text{-}CH_3O\text{-}C_6H_4$	H	H	5.34
$m\text{-}CH_3O\text{-}C_6H_4$	H	H	4.23
C_6H_5	C_6H_5	H	0.85

phosphoric, tartaric, succinic, citric, and maleic acids (Fig. 10-6). Hydrochloric acid is a monobasic acid; it has one proton and therefore reacts with one molecule of base. The others are dibasic acids (sulfuric, tartaric, succinic, and maleic) and tribasic acids (citric and phosphoric). The aqueous solution of the amine salt will have a characteristic pH that will vary depending on the acid used. The pH will be acidic when a strong mineral acid is used to prepare the salt or weakly acidic or neutral if a weak organic acid is used. Since the amine is converted to a water-soluble salt by the action of the acid, it is reasonable to assume that the addition of a base to the salt would result in liberation of the free amine, which in turn may precipitate. This is a chemical incompatibility that could be quite important when drugs are mixed.

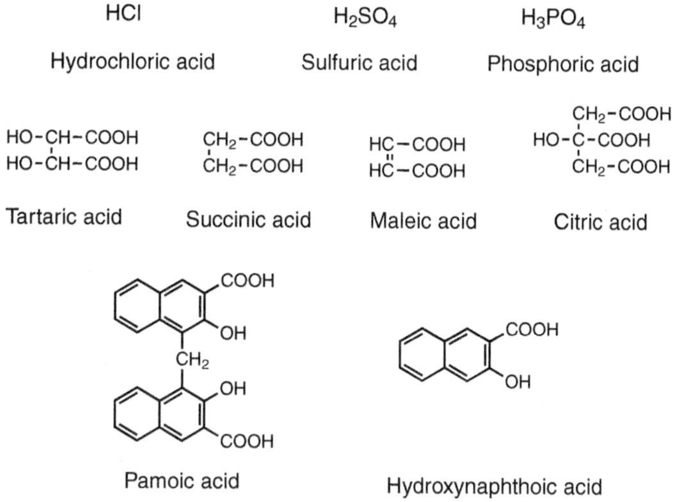

HCl H_2SO_4 H_3PO_4

Hydrochloric acid   Sulfuric acid   Phosphoric acid

$$HO-CH-COOH$$
$$HO-CH-COOH$$

$$CH_2-COOH$$
$$CH_2-COOH$$

$$HC-COOH$$
$$HC-COOH$$

$$CH_2-COOH$$
$$HO-C-COOH$$
$$CH_2-COOH$$

Tartaric acid   Succinic acid   Maleic acid   Citric acid

Pamoic acid   Hydroxynaphthoic acid

FIGURE 10-6. Structure of common acids used to prepare salts of basic amines.

Included in Figure 10-6 are two additional commonly used acids, pamoic and hydroxynaphthoic acid. These acids are commonly used in medicinal chemistry to form amine salts that are water-insoluble (in other words, salts that will not dissociate). This property is used to good advantage in that it prevents a drug from being absorbed and thus keeps the drug in the intestinal tract.

■ **METABOLISM.** Many metabolic routes are available for handling amines in the body, some of which are illustrated in Figure 10-7. A common reaction that secondary and tertiary amines undergo is dealkylation. In the dealkylation reaction, the alkyl group is lost as an aldehyde or ketone and the amine is converted from a tertiary amine to a secondary amine and finally to a primary amine. This reaction usually occurs when the amine is substituted with small alkyl groups such as a methyl, ethyl, or propyl group. An example of a drug metabolized by a dealkylation

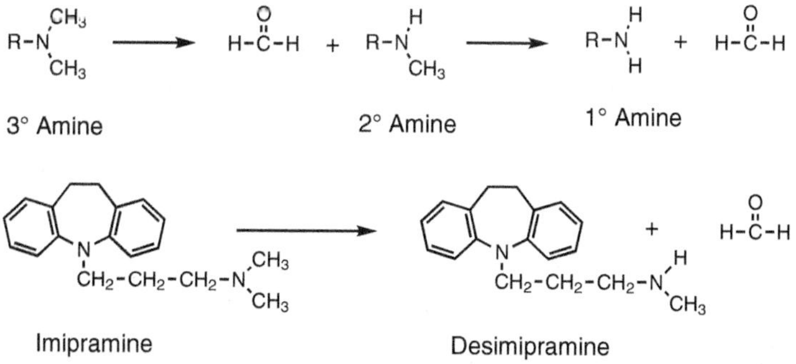

3° Amine   2° Amine   1° Amine

Imipramine   Desimipramine

FIGURE 10-7. Metabolic demethylation of tertiary and secondary amines.

reaction is imipramine, which is metabolized to desimipramine. These dealkylation reactions are commonly catalyzed by members of the cytochrome P450 family of enzymes.

Primary alkyl amines can also undergo a dealkylation reaction of sorts known as deamination. Here again, an aldehyde or ketone is formed along with an amine. Pyridoxal 5-phosphate may catalyze this reaction, resulting in the formation of pyridoxamine. For this reaction to occur, a carbon bonded to the nitrogen must be substituted with at least one hydrogen. The enzymes most commonly found that catalyze deamination reactions are monoamine oxidase (MAO) and diamine oxidase (DAO). An example of an MAO-catalyzed reaction is the deamination of norepinephrine, as shown in Figure 10-8. MAO is not a cytochrome P450 enzyme,

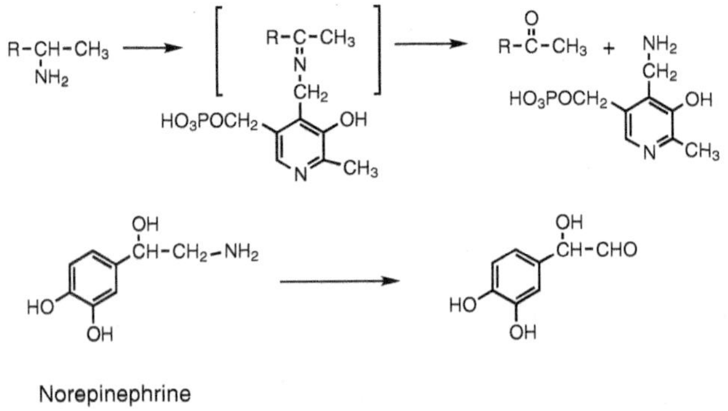

FIGURE 10-8. Metabolic deamination of a primary amine catalyzed by pyridoxal phosphate.

although under some circumstances primary amines may undergo a CYP450-catalyzed dealkylation.

Tertiary acyclic and cyclic amines and some secondary acyclic and cyclic amines can also undergo oxidation reactions catalyzed by CYP450 isoforms and microsomal flavin-containing mono-oxygenase (FMO). N-oxidation of a tertiary amine leads to an N-oxide as shown in Figure 10-9.

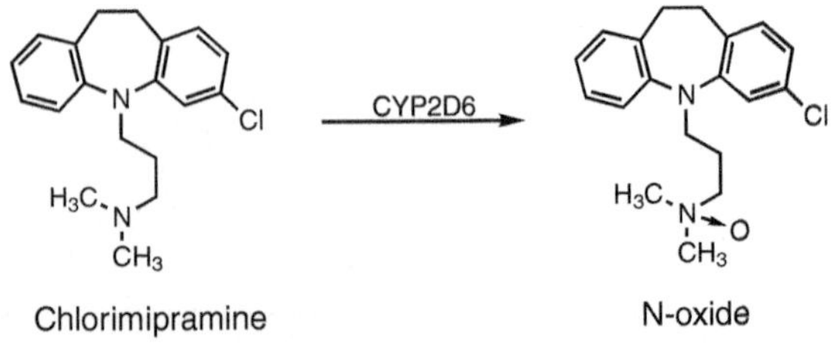

Chlorimipramine   N-oxide

FIGURE 10-9. Nitrogen oxidation of a teritiay amine leading to the N-oxide.

A minor metabolic route open to amines is the methylation reaction. An important example of the methylation reaction is the biosynthesis of epinephrine from norepinephrine catalyzed by a variety of methyltransferases including the enzyme phenylethanolamine-N-methyltransferase (PNMT) and requiring the cofactor S-adenosylmethionine (SAM) (Fig. 10-10). Methylation is considered a phase 2 conjugation reaction in which lipophilicity actually increases.

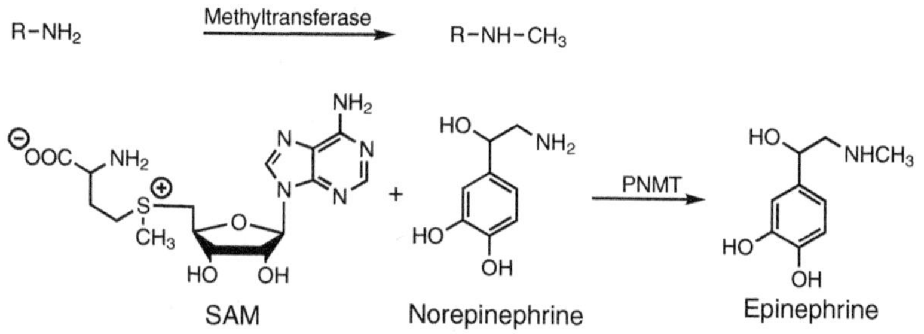

FIGURE 10-10. Metabolic methylation of an amine.

Quite important to the metabolism of primary and secondary, and a small number of tertiary, amines are the more common phase 2 conjugation reactions (see Appendix C). Amines can be conjugated with glucuronic acid to give glucuronides. The glucuronide of an amine is a **mixed acetal** functional group. Conjugation of amines with sulfuric acid gives rise to sulfate conjugates. Both glucuronide and sulfate conjugates exhibit a significant increase in water solubility. Amines, especially primary aryl amines, may also be acetylated by acetyl CoA to give a compound that usually shows a decrease in water solubility (Fig. 10-11).

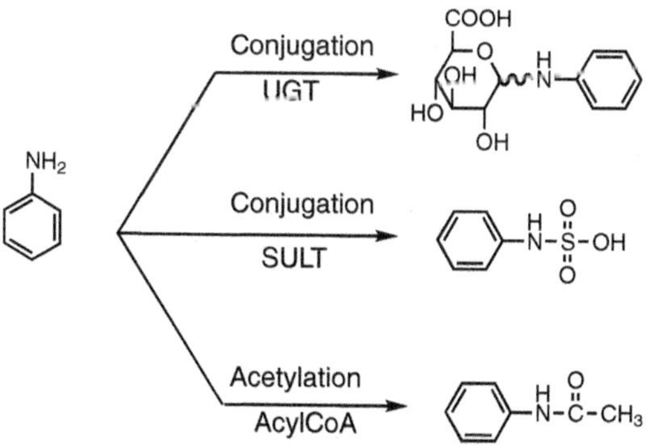

FIGURE 10-11. Metabolic conjugation of a primary amines with glucuronic acid, sulfuric acid, and acetyl coenzyme A (phase 2 conjugations).

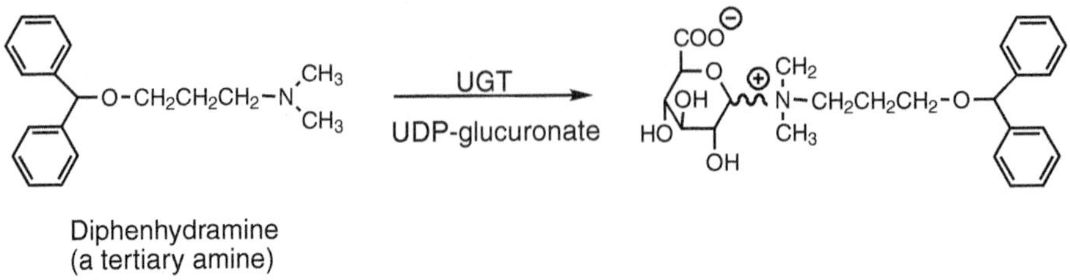

Diphenhydramine
(a tertiary amine)

FIGURE 10-12. Glucuronidation of diphenhydramine.

A less common phase 2 glucuronidation has been reported for a small number of tertiary amines and is illustrated in Figure 10-12. The resulting quaternary amine has improved water solubility and is quite unstable. As a result these conjugates often are not isolated, but rather the unconjugated parent drug is recovered in the urine or stools. These conjugated quaternary ammonium salts differ from those to be discussed in the next section in that they are salts of a mixed acetal which is the cause for the instability.

QUATERNARY AMMONIUM SALTS

Special amine derivatives with unique properties are the quaternary ammonium salts.

■ **NOMENCLATURE.** While the reaction of primary, secondary, or tertiary amines with acid leads to the formation of the respective ammonium salts, these reactions can be reversed by treatment with base, regenerating the initial amines (Fig. 10-13). The quaternary ammonium salts we wish to consider here are those compounds in which the nitrogen is bound to four carbon atoms through covalent bonds.

The quaternary ammonium salts are stable compounds that are not converted to amines by treatment with base. The nitrogen-carbon bonds may be alkyl bonds, aryl bonds, or a mixture of alkyl-aryl bonds. The nomenclature is derived by naming the organic substituents, followed by the word "ammonium" and then the particular salt that is present. An example is the compound tetraethyl ammonium (TEA) sulfate:

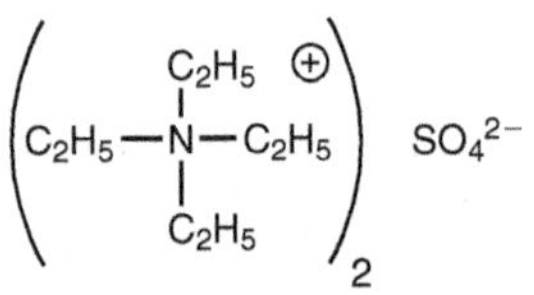

$$\left(\begin{array}{c} \overset{C_2H_5}{\underset{C_2H_5}{\overset{\oplus}{C_2H_5-N-C_2H_5}}} \end{array} \right)_2 SO_4^{2-}$$

TEA sulfate

■ **PHYSICAL-CHEMICAL PROPERTIES.** Although the ammonium salts formed from primary, secondary, and tertiary amines are reversible, as shown in Figure 10-13, this is not true of quaternary ammonium salts. These salts are relatively stable and require considerable energy to break the carbon-nitrogen bond. The quaternary

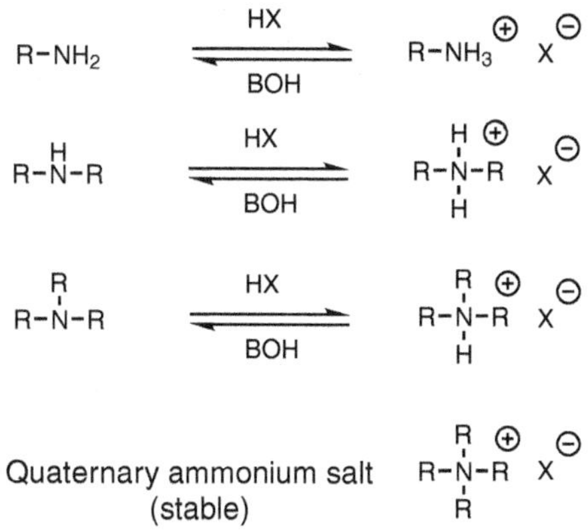

FIGURE 10-13. Ammonium salt formation and comparison with a quaternary ammonium salt.

ammonium salts are ionic compounds that, if the salt is capable of dissociation in water, exhibit significant water solubility. Ion-dipole bonding to water of the quaternary ammonium has the potential of dissolving 20 to 30 carbon atoms. Most of the quaternary ammonium salts commonly seen in pharmacy are water-soluble.

■ **METABOLISM.** There is no special metabolism of quaternary ammonium salts that the student need be familiar with.

Case Study 10.1

RK is a 73-year-old male who has been diagnosed with acute nonlymphocytic leukemia. His medical history includes congestive heart failure (CHF) and a previous myocardial infarction that nearly took his life. RK's oncologist is contemplating chemotherapy with one of the two anthracycline-based anticancer agents drawn below, but is concerned because she is fully aware that anthracycline anticancer drugs can induce potentially fatal cardiotoxicity that presents as drug-resistant CHF.

You understand that the mechanism of acute anthracycline cardiotoxicity includes the generation of highly damaging free radicals (especially hydroxyl radical, ˙OH) in the myocardium. This cytotoxic radical is formed as a byproduct of the reduction of the quinone ring (marked with a **Q**) to the hydroquinone. The more the quinone oxygen atoms can be stabilized, the more resistant to metabolism and the lower the risk of free radical-induced cardiac damage.

1. Assuming that either drug would provide therapeutic benefit to this cancer patient, which one would be less likely to damage his vulnerable heart, and why?

(case study continues on page 60)

Case Study 10.1 (continued)

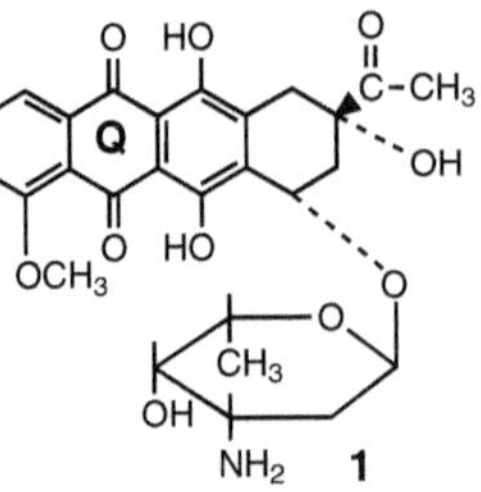

Focus your attention on anticancer agent **2**. This drug is administered IV in hydrochloride salt form.

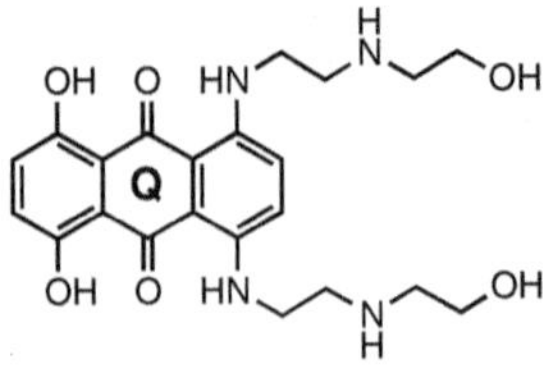

2. Which of the two secondary amines would be the preferential site for protonation by hydrochloric acid, and why (amine choices shown on only one arm of the drug)?

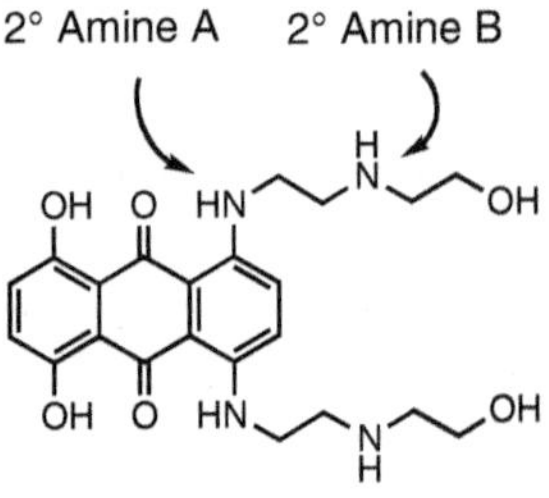

Case Study 10.2

You are a P-4 student serving on your school's curriculum committee. During a recent meeting, the student representing the P-1 class suggests that the committee consider eliminating the course in organic functional groups because she feels it is unimportant to pharmacy practice. A faculty member on the committee then

(case study continues on page 61)

Case Study 10.2 (continued)

challenges you to defend the course by asking you to explain the importance of the α-amino functional group on ampicillin. He reminds you that benzylpenicillin decomposes in acid as shown below.

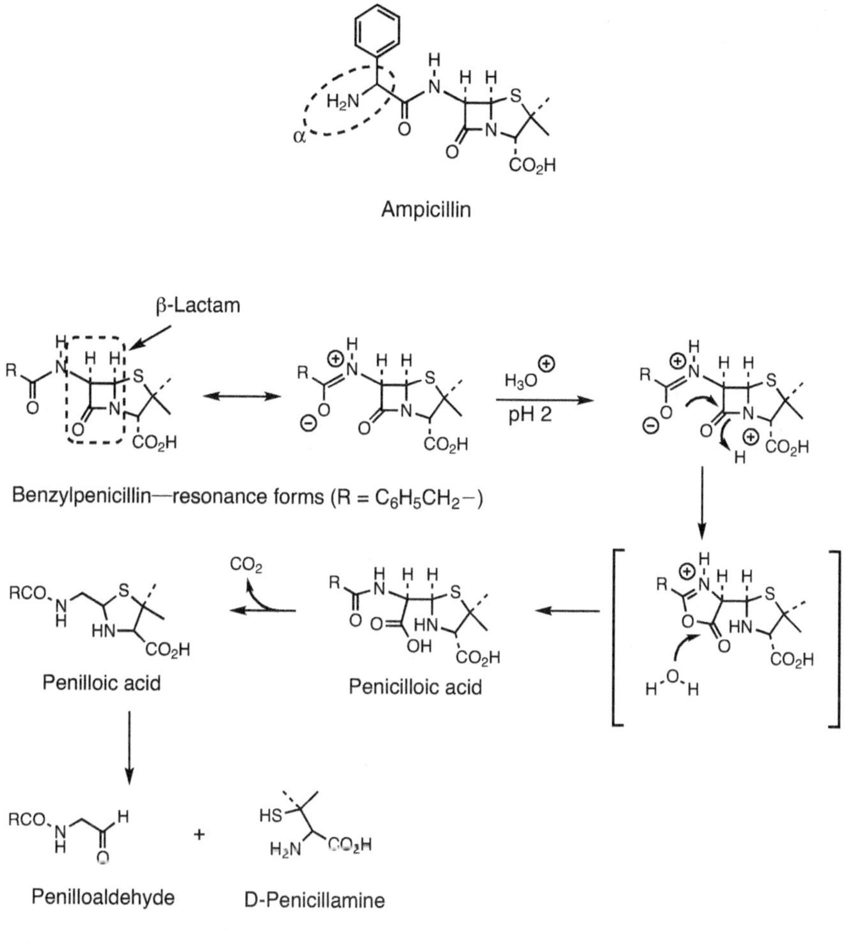
α
Ampicillin
β-Lactam
Benzylpenicillin—resonance forms (R = $C_6H_5CH_2-$)
H_3O^+
pH 2
CO_2
Penilloic acid
Penicilloic acid
Penilloaldehyde
D-Penicillamine

Instability of benzylpenicillin in acid.

Carboxylic Acids

11

■ **NOMENCLATURE.** A carboxylic acid is a molecule that contains a characteristic carboxyl group to which is attached a hydrogen, alkyl, aryl, or heterocyclic substituent. The common nomenclature of the carboxylic acids is used more often than with most other functional groups, probably because of the wide variety of carboxylic acids found in nature and the fact that they were named before the chemistry of the molecules was understood. Even without branching of the alkyl chains, this nomenclature becomes difficult to remember, with such uncommon names as caproic (C_6), caprylic (C_8), capric (C_{10}), and lauric (C_{12}) acids. The official nomenclature returns to the use of the hydrocarbon names such as methane, ethane, propane, butane, and pentane. As with all IUPAC nomenclature, the longest continuous chain containing the functional group, in this case the carboxyl group, is chosen as the base unit. The hydrocarbon name is used, the "e" is dropped and replaced with "oic," which signifies a carboxyl group, and this is followed by the word "acid." This is illustrated in Figure 11-1.

■ **NOMENCLATURE—BIOLOGICALLY IMPORTANT CARBOXYLIC ACIDS.** The student should be familiar with a number of biologically significant carboxylic acids related to drug actions and nutrition. Mevalonic acid, one such compound, is a key

Structure	Common name	IUPAC name
O ‖ H–C–OH	Formic acid	Methan<u>oic</u> acid
O ‖ CH₃–C–OH	Acetic acid (Vinegar)	Ethan<u>oic</u> acid
O ‖ CH₃–CH₂–C–OH	Propionic acid	Propan<u>oic</u> acid
O ‖ CH₃–CH₂–CH₂–CH₂–CH₂–C–OH	Caproic acid	Hexan<u>oic</u> acid
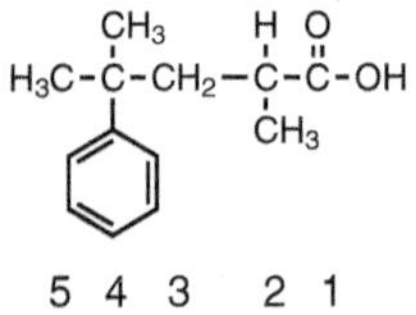 CH₃ H O H₃C–C–CH₂–C–C–OH ⬡ CH₃	2,4-Dimethyl-4-phenylpentan<u>oic</u> acid	

5 4 3   2 1

FIGURE 11-1. Examples of Common and Official (IUPAC) nomenclature for carboxylic acids.

intermediate in the biosynthesis of cholesterol, which itself serves as the precursor to most of the steroid hormones in the human body.

Mevalonic acid
(3,5-Dihydroxy-3-
methylpentanoic acid)

Squalene ----> Steroids
(Cholesterol)

Important in human nutrition are the natural occurring carboxylic acids commonly referred to as fatty acids. The fatty acid terminology relates to the physicochemical property of being quite fat soluble. Included within this group are lauric, myristic, palmitic, and stearic acid (Table 11-1). It should be noted that these acids all have an even number of carbons which relate to their common biosynthetic pathway in which two carbon acetate units are linked together to form the natural occurring fatty acids. In addition, the above acids are all saturated fatty acids indicating no multiple bonds are present and that all the carbons, with the exception of the carboxylic acid group, are fully saturated with hydrogen. Palmitic and stearic acids are the most abundant of the saturated fatty acids.

A second group of fatty acids are the monounsaturated fatty acids. The most common members of this class of agents are palmitoleic acid and oleic acid. A common feature of the monounsaturated fatty acids is that the double bond is usually found at the nine position (Δ^9) and is "*cis*" in stereochemistry (**Z-configuration**). Natural

Table 11-1. BOILING POINTS (BP)/MELTING POINTS (MP) AND WATER SOLUBILITY OF COMMON ORGANIC ACIDS

CARBOXYLIC ACID	$R-\overset{O}{\overset{\|}{C}}-OH$	bp/mp °C	SOLUBILITY (g/100g H_2O)	(g/100g EtOH)
Formic	H	100.5	∞	∞
Acetic	CH_3	118.0	∞	∞
Propionic	CH_3CH_2	141.0	∞	∞
Butyric	$CH_3(CH_2)_2$	164.0	∞	∞
Pentanoic	$CH_3(CH_2)_3$	187.0	3.7	Soluble
Hexanoic	$CH_3(CH_2)_4$	205.0	1.0	Soluble
Benzoic	C_6H_5	250.0	0.34	Soluble
Decanoic	$CH_3(CH_2)_8$	31.4	0.015	Soluble
Lauric	$CH_3(CH_2)_{10}$	44.0	Insoluble	100.0
Myristic	$CH_3(CH_2)_{12}$	58.5	Insoluble	Soluble
Palmitic	$CH_3(CH_2)_{14}$	63–64	Insoluble	Sparingly
Stearic	$CH_3(CH_2)_{16}$	69–70	Insoluble	5.0

occurring fatty acids have a *"cis"* stereochemistry while the presence of a *"trans"* double bond (**E-configuration**) arises during food processing and is unnatural.

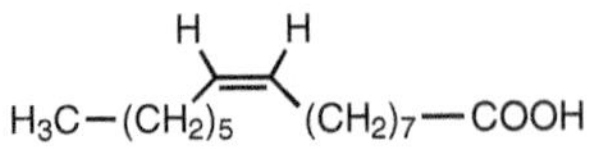

Palmitoleic acid

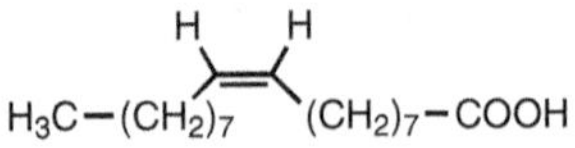

Oleic acid

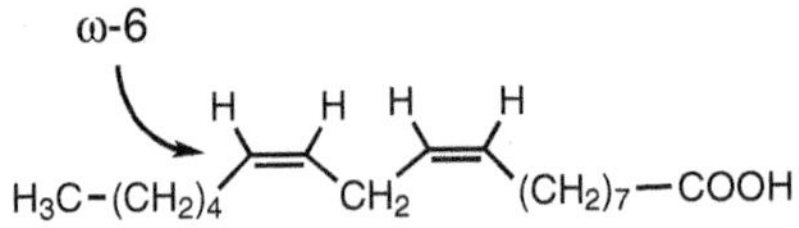

Linoleic acid

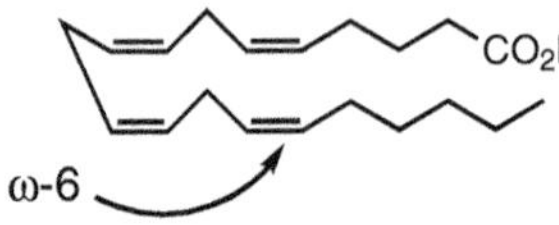

Arachidonic acid

A third group of fatty acids are the polyunsaturated fatty acids. By definition, polyunsaturated suggests two or more double bonds. The most common polyunsaturated fatty acids are linolenic, linoleic, and arachidonic acid which are also known as the omega fatty acids (the first is ω-3 and the latter two are ω-6). The omega nomenclature indicates that a double bond is found either three carbons from the terminal methyl group or six carbons from the terminal methyl group, respectively. Linoleic and linolenic acid are commonly referred to as the "essential

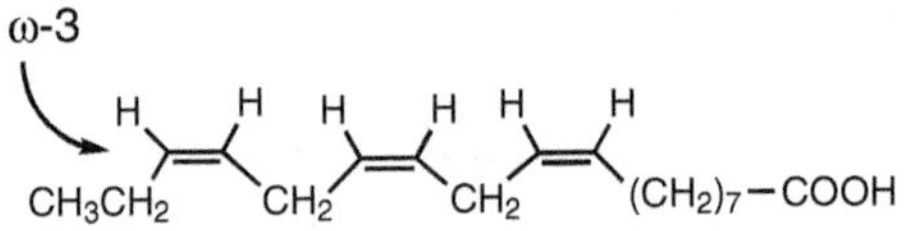

Linolenic acid

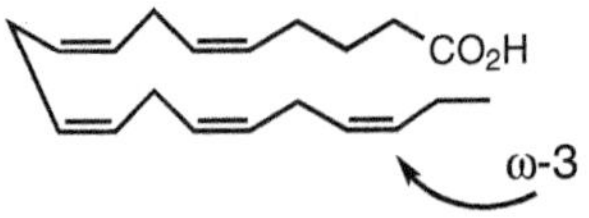

Eicosapentaenoic acid (EPA)

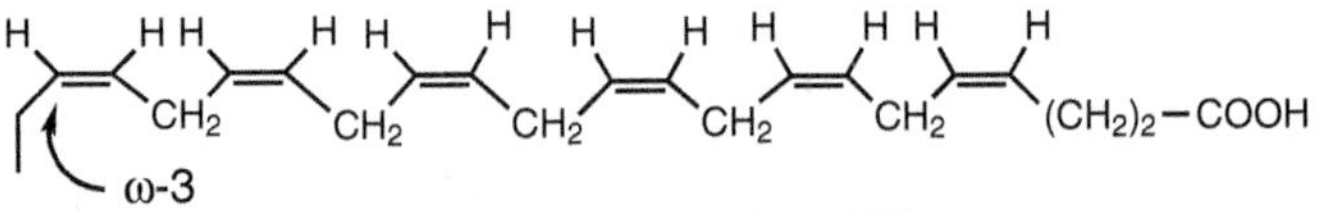

Docosahexaenoic acid (DHA)

fatty acids" in that they are essential for the synthesis of cell membranes as well as other functions in the body. Arachidonic acid is a key intermediate in the biosynthesis of the prostaglandin, prostacyclin, and thromboxane hormones (Fig. 11-2). Most recently, several dietary fish oils have been identified as having significant effects in reducing coronary artery disease. Examples of important fish oils are EPA (a precursor to prostaglandin-3) and DHA.

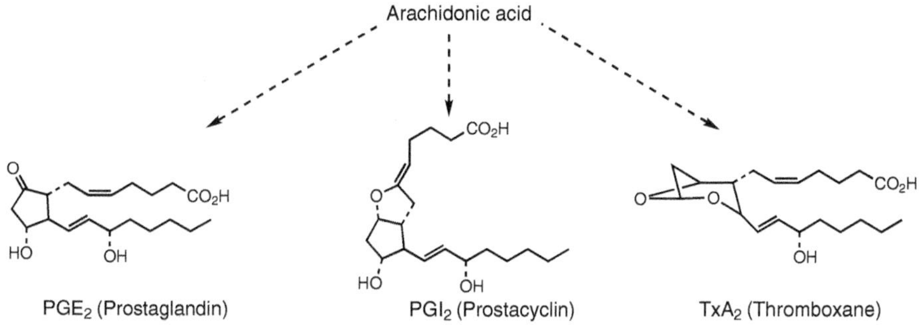

FIGURE 11-2. Biosynthesis of prostaglandins, prostacyclins, and thromboxanes from arachidonic acid.

▪ **PHYSICAL-CHEMICAL PROPERTIES.** The carboxylic acid functional group consists of a carbonyl and a hydroxyl group; both, when taken individually, are polar groups that can hydrogen bond. The hydrogen of the -OH can hydrogen bond to either of the oxygen groups in another carboxyl function (Fig. 11-3). The amount and strength of hydrogen bonding in the case of a carboxylic acid are greater than in the case of alcohols or phenols because of the greater acidity of the carboxylic acid and because of the additional sites of bonding. From this discussion, one could predict that carboxylic acids are high-boiling liquids and solids. If the carboxyl can strongly hydrogen bond to itself, then it is reasonable to predict that the carboxyl group can hydrogen bond to water, resulting in water solubility. In Table 11-1, the effect of the strong intermolecular hydrogen bonding can be seen by examining the boiling points of several of the carboxylic acids, while the strong hydrogen bonding to water is demonstrated by the solubility of the carboxylic acids in water. Once again, as the lipophilic hydrocarbon chain length increases, the water solubility decreases drastically. A carboxyl group will solubilize (1% or greater concentration) approximately five carbon atoms.

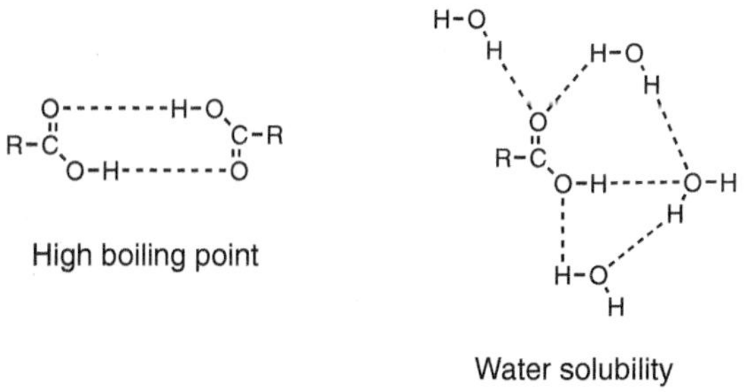

FIGURE 11-3. Intermolecular bonding of carboxylic acids to themselves and to water.

Another solvent important in pharmacy is ethanol. Ethanol has both a hydrophilic and lipophilic portion, and bonding between an organic molecule and ethanol therefore may involve both dipole-dipole bonding and van der Waals bonding (Fig. 11-4).

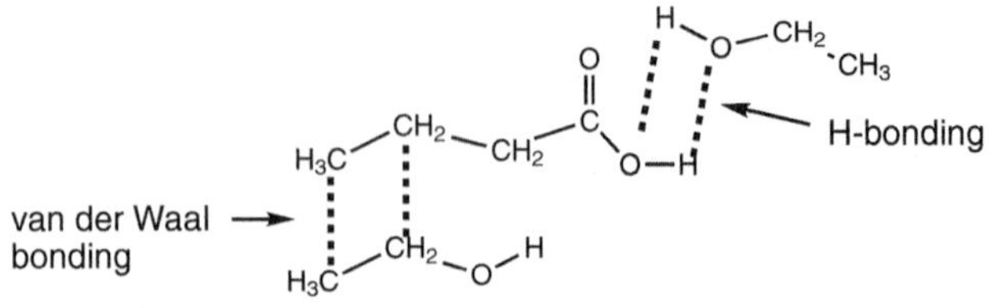

FIGURE 11-4. Chemical bonding between butyric acid and ethanol.

It is not surprising, then, that the solubility of the carboxylic acids is much greater in ethanol than it is in water. Although pure ethanol cannot be used internally, ethanol-water combinations can, and they greatly increase the solution potential of many drugs.

Turning now to an extremely important property of the carboxylic acids, their acidic property, one sees the familiar dissociation of a carboxylic acid (giving up a proton) shown in Table 11-2. This dissociation, by definition, makes the group an acid.

From general chemistry it will be recalled that the strength of an acid depends on the concentration of protons in solution, which depends on dissociation. The value of K_1 and K_{-1} in turn depends on the stability of the carboxylate anion in relation to the undissociated carboxylic acid. In other words, if we are considering two acids, acid 1 (in which the carboxylate anion is unstable) and acid 2 (in which the carboxylate anion is stable), acid 2, with the more stable carboxylate, will dissociate to a greater extent, giving up a higher concentration of protons, and therefore is a stronger acid. It has been found that the nature of the R-group *does* influence the stability of the carboxylate anion, and it does so in the following manner: if R is an electron donor group, as shown in Table 11-2, it will destabilize the carboxylate anion and thus decrease the acidity (this is represented by the dissociation arrows). To understand how this comes about, one must look at the carboxylate anion. This anion is stabilized by resonance, with the negative charge not remaining fixed on the oxygen but instead being spread across the oxygen-carbon-oxygen. Now, if electrons are pushed toward a region already high in electron density, repulsion occurs. This is an unfavorable situation. In the nonionic carboxylic acid form, resonance stabilization is not occurring to the same extent and the problem is reduced. Therefore, in Example 1, the nonionic form is more stable than the ionic form. In Example 2, the opposite effect is considered: electron withdrawal by the R-group. Reducing electron density around the carbonyl carbon should increase the ease of resonance stabilization, in turn increasing the stability of the carboxylate anion. Considering Example 2 in relationship to Example 1, one would predict that acid 2 would be more acidic than acid 1. Table 11-2 has examples of compounds that fit this description. The methyl group is an electron donor that reduces the acidity with respect to that of formic acid, while the phenyl can be considered an electron sink or, with respect to alkyl acids, an electron-withdrawing group; therefore, benzoic acid is a stronger acid than acetic acid. The addition of halogens to an alkyl changes the nature of the alkyl. In chloroacetic acid, the chloride, being electronegative, pulls electrons away from the carbon, which in turn pulls electrons away from the carbonyl. This effect is quite strong, as is seen in

Table 11-2. DISSOCIATION CONSTANTS AND pK$_a$ VALUES IN WATER OF COMMON CARBOXYLIC ACIDS

$$R-\overset{\overset{O}{\|}}{C}-OH + H_2O \rightleftharpoons H_3O^{\oplus} + R-\overset{\overset{O}{\|}}{C}-O^{\ominus} \longleftrightarrow R-C\overset{O}{\underset{O}{\diagdown}}{}^{\ominus}$$

Example 1: $R\rightarrow\overset{\overset{O}{\|}}{C}-OH + H_2O \rightleftharpoons H_3O^{\oplus} + R\rightarrow\overset{\overset{O}{\|}}{C}-O^{\ominus}$

Example 2: $R\leftarrow\overset{\overset{O}{\|}}{C}-OH + H_2O \rightleftharpoons H_3O^{\oplus} + R\leftarrow\overset{\overset{O}{\|}}{C}-O^{\ominus}$

$R-\overset{\overset{O}{\|}}{C}-OH$	Dissociation Constant (K$_a$ and pK$_a$)	
	K$_a$ (in water)	pK$_a$
H	17.7×10^{-5}	3.75
CH_3	1.75×10^{-5}	4.76
$Cl-CH_2$	1.36×10^{-3}	2.87
Cl_2CH	5.53×10^{-2}	1.26
Cl_3C	2.32×10^{-1}	0.64
C_6H_5	6.30×10^{-5}	4.21
p-CH_3-C_6H_4	4.20×10^{-5}	4.38
m-CH_3-C_6H_4	5.40×10^{-5}	4.27
P-NO_2-C_6H_4	3.60×10^{-4}	3.44
m-NO_2-C_6H_4	3.20×10^{-4}	3.50

the K$_a$. This electron-withdrawing effect continues to increase as the number of halogens increases to give a strong carboxylic acid, trichloroacetic acid.

As discussed earlier for phenols and aromatic amines, substitution on the aromatic ring of benzoic acid will influence acidity. Ortho substitution is not always predictable, but in most cases the acidity of the acid is increased by ortho substitution. Meta and para substitutions are predictable. Substitution on the benzene ring with an electron-releasing group decreases acidity. If this substituent is para, the decrease in acidity with respect to benzoic acid will be greater than if the substituent is meta. If the substituent is an electron-withdrawing group, the acidity of the acid will increase. The greatest increase is observed when the substituent is para. One should recall that this is the same trend seen for substituted phenols.

Another property of carboxylic acids is their reactivity toward base. Carboxylic acids will react with a base to give a salt, as shown in Table 11-3. If one is considering water solubility, the interaction of a salt with water through dipole-ion bonding is much stronger than dipole-dipole interaction of the acid. Therefore, a

Table 11-3. SOLUBILITY PROPERTIES OF SODIUM SALTS OF COMMON ORGANIC ACIDS

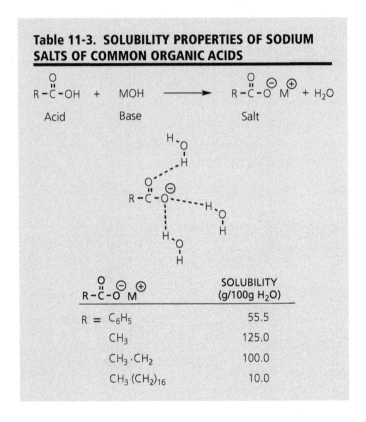

$R-\overset{O}{\overset{\|}{C}}-O^{\ominus}\ M^{\oplus}$	SOLUBILITY (g/100g H_2O)
R = C_6H_5	55.5
CH_3	125.0
$CH_3 \cdot CH_2$	100.0
$CH_3(CH_2)_{16}$	10.0

considerable increase in water solubility should and does occur. The same point must be made here as was made with phenol and amine salts: the salt must be able to dissociate in order to dissolve in water. Salts formed from carboxylic acids and sodium, potassium, or ammonium hydroxide show a great increase in water solubility. Salts formed with heavy metals tend to be relatively insoluble. Examples of such insoluble salts are the heavy metal salts (e.g., calcium, magnesium, zinc, aluminium) of carboxylic acids. When salts of carboxylic acids dissolve in water, a characteristic alkaline pH is common. With sodium and potassium salts, the pH is generally quite high. As with other salts, if acid is now added to this solution, one can reverse the carboxylic acid-base reaction and regenerate the carboxylic acid. The free acid is less soluble than was the salt, and precipitation may result. This is an important chemical incompatibility that one should keep in mind when dealing with water-soluble carboxylate salts. In summary, amines and carboxylic acids are common functional groups found in drugs. These groups have a potentiating effect on solubility, and both groups can form salts that, if capable of dissociation, will greatly increase water solubility.

■ **METABOLISM.** The metabolism of the carboxylic acids is relatively simple. Carboxylic acids can undergo a variety of conjugation reactions (phase 2 metabolism; see Appendix C). They can conjugate with UDPGA (the activated form of glucuronic acid) in the presence of UGT to form glucuronides and also with amino acids (Fig. 11-5). Activation of the fatty acid by acetyl CoA followed by transacetylation with glycine or glutamine leads to the amino acid conjugates.

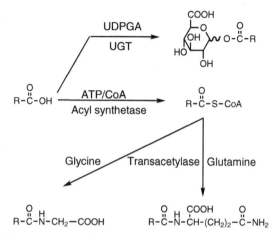

FIGURE 11-5. Metabolic conjugation of carboxylic acids.

Another common type of metabolism of alkyl carboxylic acids is oxidation beta to the carboxyl group. This is a common reaction in the metabolism of fatty acids. The reaction proceeds through a sequence in which the carboxyl group is bound to coenzyme A (CoA). The bound acid is oxidized to enoyl CoA, hydrated to β-hydroxyacetyl CoA, oxidized to β-ketoacyl CoA, and finally cleaved to the shortened carboxylic acid plus acetic acid, as shown in Figure 11-6. This is a phase 1 metabolism.

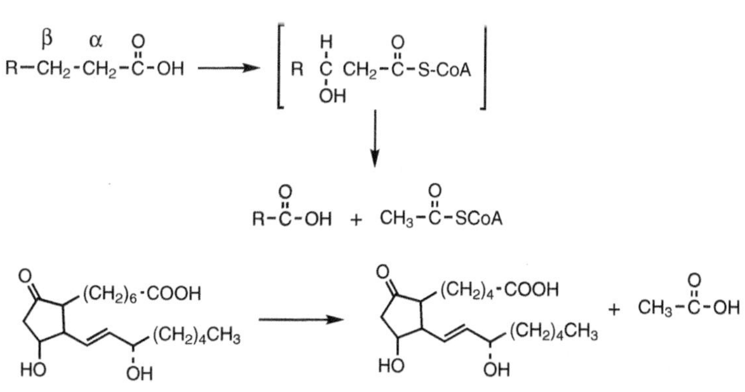

FIGURE 11-6. Beta oxidation of alkyl carboxylic acids.

Case Study 11.1

KF is a 38 year-old driver for *East Coast Corridor*, a company offering narrated bus tours of Washington, D.C., New York City, and all points in between. The company is known for its well-informed staff and friendly service, which has made it a favorite of high schools sponsoring senior trips to the nation's capital. KF is regularly out on the road from Monday through Friday but, being a devout family man, he is always home in the evenings and on weekends.

KF's 5-year-old daughter wants to adopt a stray cat she has been feeding for the past several weeks and, despite being allergic to these animals, KF just cannot say no to his "best girl." He knows that many antihistamines can cause drowsiness, which would be a dangerous (as opposed to just annoying) side effect in his line of work. He turns to you, his trusted family pharmacist, to guide him toward the best therapeutic solution.

Recognizing that antihistamines capable of forming a zwitterion (an internal salt) are very often nonsedative, you study the three structural choices shown below before making a recommendation. Which of these three agents would be appropriate for KF? What's the chemical basis for your decision?

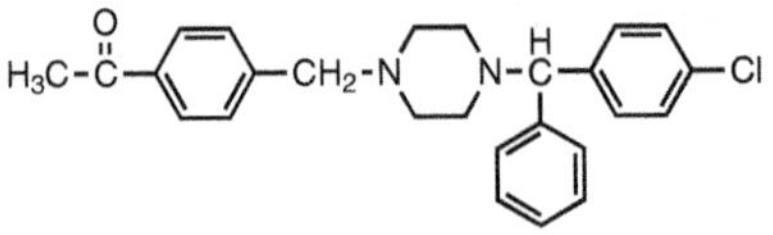

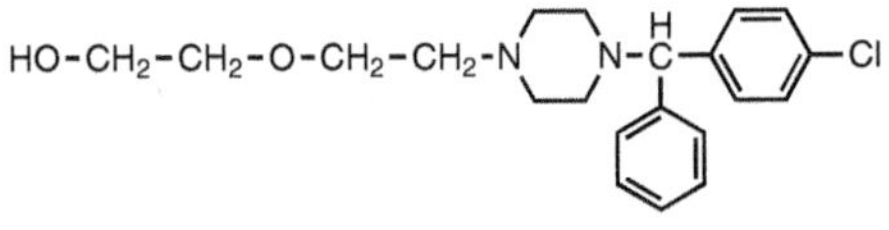

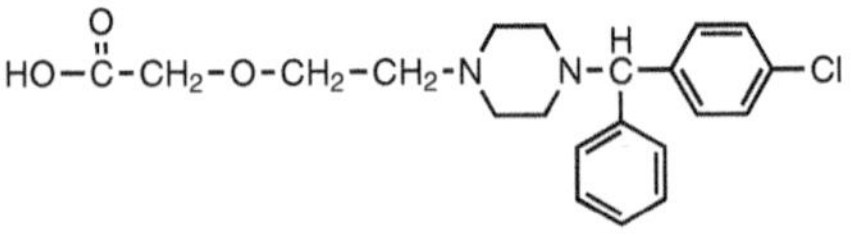

Case Study 11.2

ET is a 67-year-old woman with hypertension. ET is retired after 50 years of working as a janitor in a large paint manufacturing company. Her years of inhaling paint fumes and cleaning solvents left her with compromised liver function. ET has a family history of Wilson disease and although asymptomatic the disease was prophylactically treated with penicillamine when she was 30 years old. As a result she developed a sulfhydryl-induced maculopapular rash causing the discontinuation of the penicillamine. She was then switched to zinc acetate and continues to be asymptomatic.

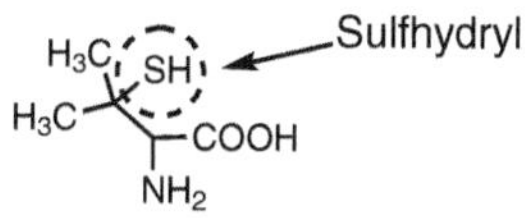

Penicillamine

ET's hypertension has become uncontrollable on a thiazide diuretic and her physician wants to add an angiotensin-converting enzyme (ACE) inhibitor to her regimen. You recall from your days in pharmacy school that the ACE inhibitors all contain one or more carboxylic acid functional groups as key to their binding to both the zinc ion and the cationic amino group of the arginine in the catalytic site.

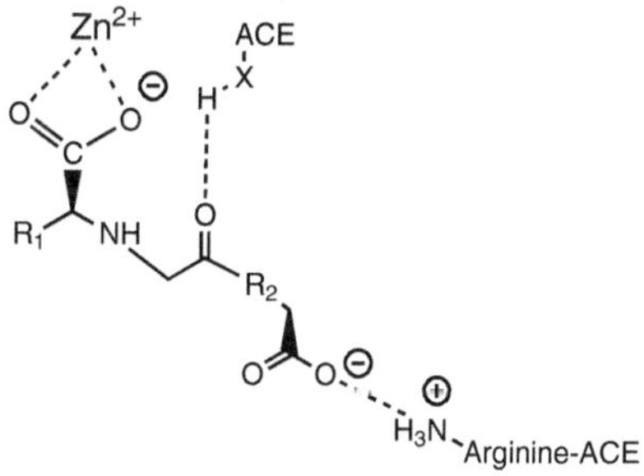

A model of inhibitor binding to ACE

(case study continues on page 72)

Case Study 11.2 (continued)

You have enalapril, captopril, and lisinopril ACE inhibitors to choose from, which would you recommend? Are you concerned about the oral bioavailability of your choice?

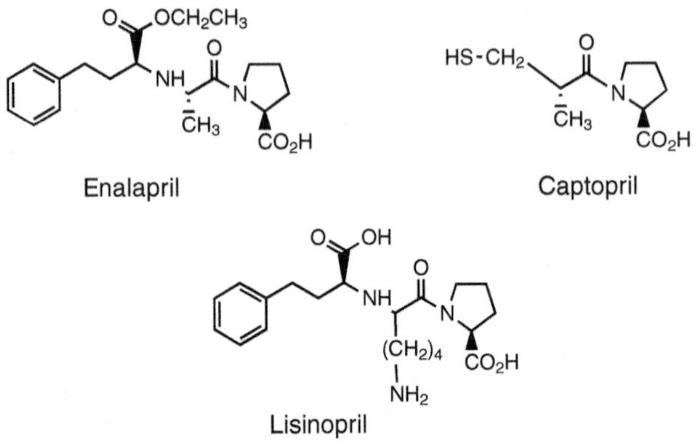

Enalapril   Captopril

Lisinopril

Before you answer you also recall that enalapril is a prodrug that requires hydrolysis of its ethyl ester in order to produce the active dicarboxylic acid metabolite, enalaprilat. Hydrolysis in vivo of the prodrug ACE inhibitors has been shown to be catalyzed in the liver by carboxylesterases instead of the more ubiquitous esterase found in the plasma (pseudocholinesterase).

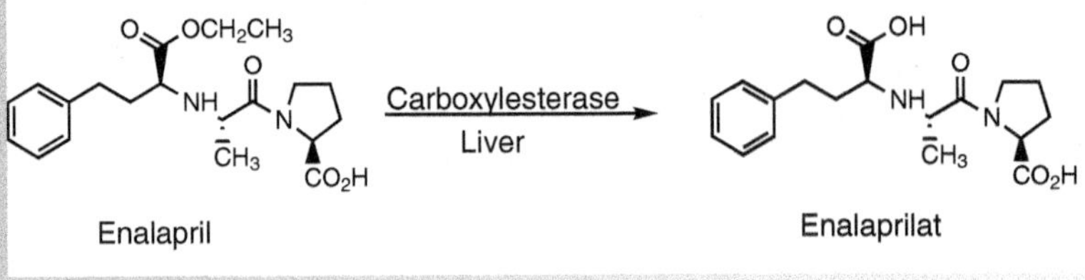

Enalapril   Enalaprilat

Functional Derivatives of Carboxylic Acids

12

In presenting the carboxylic acids, it is important to also consider several derivatives of carboxylic acids. The first to be discussed will be the esters.

ESTERS

■ **NOMENCLATURE.** The nomenclature of esters consists of combining alcohol and carboxylic acid nomenclature, either common or IUPAC nomenclature, but not a mix of both. The name of the alcohol radical comes first, followed by a space, and then the name of the acid. To show that it is a functional derivative of an acid, the "ic" ending of the acid is dropped and replaced by "ate." Examples are shown in Figure 12-1. If you do not remember alcohol and acid nomenclature, you should return to the appropriate sections and review this material.

A unique type of ester results from the intramolecular cyclization of an alcohol and a carboxylic acid. The resulting ester is known as a lactone (Fig. 12-2). Lactones are quite common in drug molecules and may exist with a five- (spironolactone) or six- (testolactone) membered ring up to and exceeding 14-unit rings (macrolide antibiotics such as erythromycin). The physical-chemical and metabolic properties of a lactone are the same as those of an ester.

■ **PHYSICAL-CHEMICAL PROPERTIES.** The physical properties of the esters are rather interesting and show a similarity to the ethers. In the formation of esters, a polar alcohol is combined with a polar acid to give a much less polar, low-boiling liquid. In the case of ethers, two alcohols are joined with the same decrease in polarity and boiling points. As with ethers, in the ester, the two hydroxyl groups necessary for intermolecular hydrogen bonding are destroyed, and along with this goes the loss of the intermolecular hydrogen bonding and a decrease in water solubility. Proof of this effect can be seen in Table 12-1. The boiling point of acetic acid is

$$CH_3-CH_2-\overset{\overset{\displaystyle O}{\|}}{C}-O-\overset{\overset{\displaystyle CH_3}{|}}{\underset{\underset{\displaystyle CH_3}{|}}{C}H} \qquad CH_3-\overset{\overset{\displaystyle O}{\|}}{C}-O-\overset{\overset{\displaystyle CH_3}{|}}{\underset{\underset{\displaystyle CH_3}{|}}{C}}-CH_3$$

Common: Isopropyl propion<u>ate</u>   t-Butyl acet<u>ate</u>

IUPAC : 2-Propyl propano<u>ate</u>   2-Methyl-2-propyl ethano<u>ate</u>

FIGURE 12-1. Examples of Common and Official (IUPAC) nomenclature of esters.

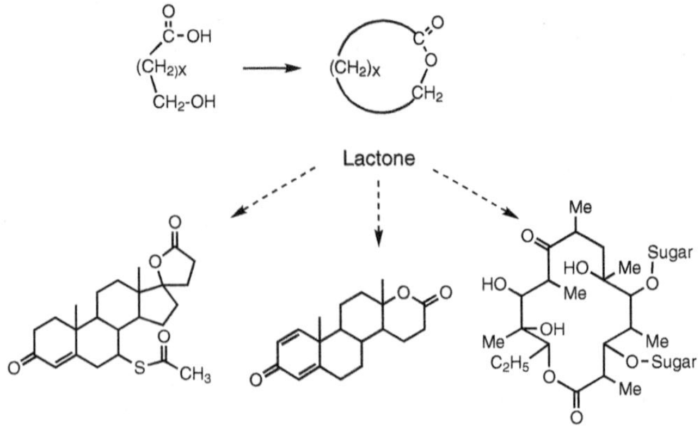

Spironolactone Testolactone Erythromycin

FIGURE 12-2. Lactone structure and examples of drug lactones.

118°, which itself is above that of many of the acetate esters. The water solubility of acids and alcohols involve hydrogen bonding from both the OH groups of the acid and alcohol as well as the OH group of water. With esters hydrogen bonding occurs between the hydrogen of water and the electron-dense oxygen of the ester carbonyl. Less potential for hydrogen bonding between the ester and water translates into less water solubility (Table 12-1). While esters are not highly water soluble, they are quite soluble in alcohol.

Table 12-1. BOILING POINTS AND WATER SOLUBILITY OF COMMON ESTERS

$R-\overset{O}{\overset{\|}{C}}-O-R'$

R	R'	BOILING POINT °C	SOLUBILITY (g/100g H_2O)
CH_3	CH_3	57.5	∞
CH_3	CH_3CH_2	77.0	10.00
CH_3CH_2	CH_3	79.7	6.25
CH_3	$CH_3CH_2CH_2$	102.0	1.60
CH_3	$CH_3CH_2CH_2CH_2$	126.0	0.83
$CH_3(CH_2)_2$	CH_3	102.0	1.67
C_6H_5	CH_3	198.0	Insoluble

An important chemical property that most esters display is the ease of hydrolysis back to the alcohol and the carboxylic acid. Esters are especially prone to base-catalyzed hydrolysis but also hydrolyze in the presence of acid and water (Fig. 12-3). What this means to medicinal chemistry is that esters are unstable in the presence of basic media in vitro and must therefore be protected from strongly alkaline conditions.

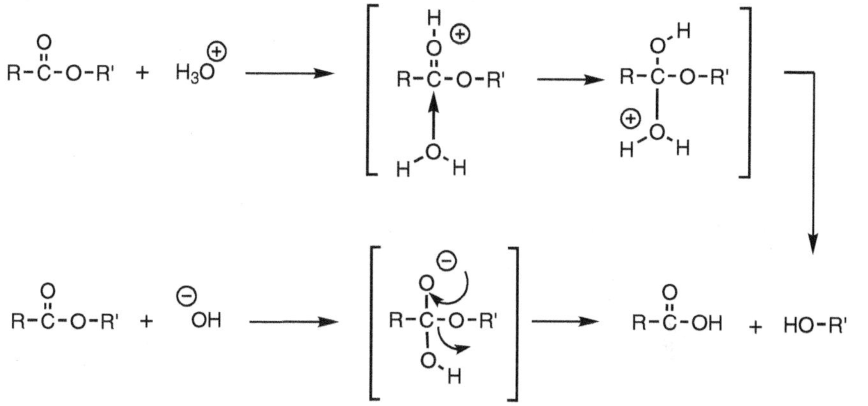

FIGURE 12-3. Acid- and base-catalyzed hydrolysis of esters.

▪ **METABOLISM.** Hydrolyzing enzymes in the body carry out hydrolysis through a base-catalyzed mechanism. It is therefore not unexpected that esters are unstable in the body and are converted to the free acid and the alcohol (Fig. 12-4). In many cases, carboxylic acids are synthetically prepared and administered as esters, even though the active drug is the acid. It is known that the acid will be regenerated metabolically.

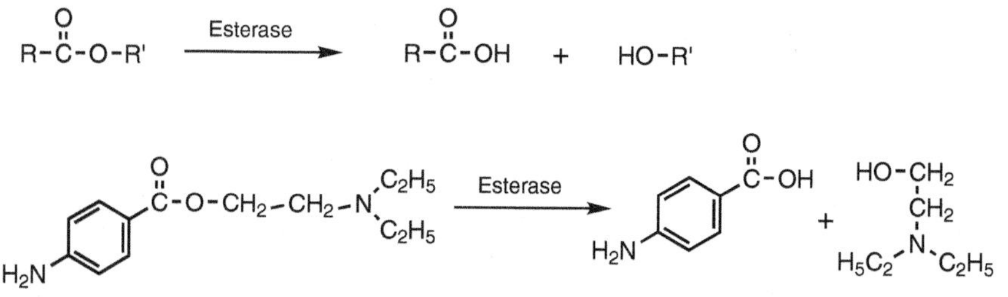

FIGURE 12-4. Metabolic hydrolysis of esters.

AMIDES

■ **NOMENCLATURE.** A second important functional derivative of the carboxylic acid is the amide. An example of the common and official nomenclature is shown in Figure 12-5. In the case of the common nomenclature, the common name of the amine followed by the common name of the acid is used. The ending "ic" of the acid is then dropped and replaced by "amide." The same approach is used for official nomenclature except that the official name of the amine and the official name of the acid are used. The "oic" ending is dropped and replaced by "amide."

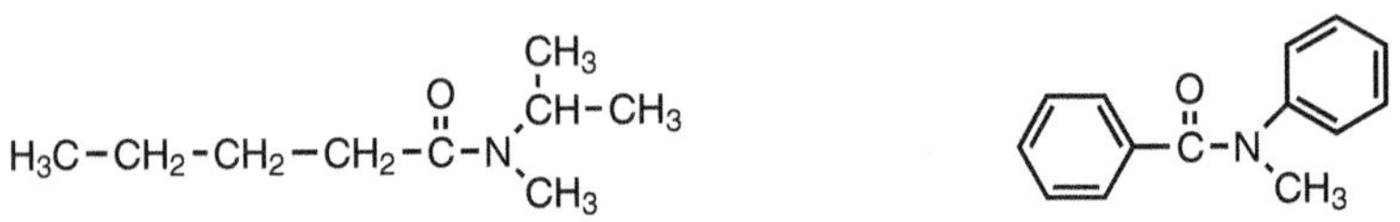

Common: N-Methyl-N-isopropylvaler<u>amide</u>   N-Methyl-N-phenylbenz<u>amide</u>

IUPAC : N-Methyl-N-2-propylpentan<u>amide</u>   N-Methyl-N-phenylbenz<u>amide</u>

FIGURE 12-5. Examples of Common and Official (IUPAC) nomenclature of amides.

A unique type of amide results from the intramolecular cyclization of an amine and a carboxylic acid. The resulting amide is known as a lactam (Fig. 12-6). As with the lactones, lactams make up the nucleus of several classes of important drugs. Probably the best-known lactam drugs are the β-lactams, which are found in the penicillin and cephalosporin antibiotics. The lactams possess physical-chemical and metabolic characteristics similar to those of the open chain amides, although with small ring compounds, such as the β-lactams, a high order of reactivity is seen.

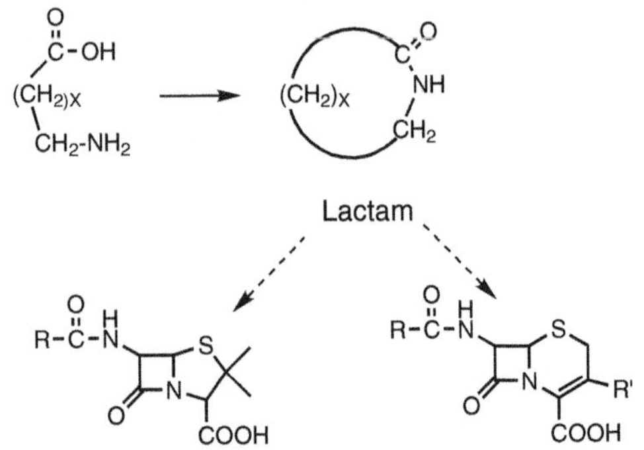

Penicillin   Cephalosporin

FIGURE 12-6. Lactam structure and examples of drug lactams.

■ **PHYSICAL-CHEMICAL PROPERTIES AND METABOLISM.** The physical properties of the amides are much different than might have been predicted after the earlier discussions of esters. Like the esters, amides result from combining a polar carboxylic acid with the weakly polar primary or secondary amine or ammonia to give the monosubstituted, disubstituted, or unsubstituted amides, respectively. The resulting amides still possess considerable polarity, as indicated by the high boiling points and water solubility (Table 12-2). These properties are quite different from those of esters. It is interesting to note that, with any series, as the substitution on the nitrogen increases, the boiling point decreases. As an example, look at formamide, N-methyl formamide, and N,N-dimethylformamide. This may be explained in part by a consideration of the resonance forms of amides, as shown in Figure 12-7. The unshared pair of electrons of the nitrogen no longer remain on the nitrogen but are spread across the nitrogen, carbon, and oxygen. This has a significant effect on the polarity of the amide. Since boiling points depend on the amount and strength of intermolecular bonding, the unsubstituted and monosubstituted amide would be expected to show strong intermolecular bonding owing to the high electron density on oxygen bonding to the hydrogens or hydrogen on the nitrogen. In the case of the disubstituted amides, both hydrogens have been replaced on the nitrogen, and intermolecular hydrogen bonding is not possible. Disubstituted amides are still capable of dipole-dipole bonding, but not through hydrogen bonding. Thus, the boiling point drops. Water solubility requires only a polar material, since the hydrogen can be supplied by the water. Both substituted and unsubstituted amides can hydrogen bond to water through the hydrogen of water and show good water solubility. As the hydrocarbon portion of the amide increases, so the lipophilic nature increases and water solubility decreases.

Table 12-2. BOILING POINTS AND WATER SOLUBILITY OF COMMON AMIDES

$$R_1-\overset{\overset{\text{O}}{\|}}{C}-N\overset{R_2}{\underset{R_3}{\cdot}}$$

R_1	R_2	R_3	BOILING POINT °C	SOLUBILITY (g/100g H_2O)
H	H	H	210	Soluble
H	CH_3	H	180	Soluble
H	CH_3	CH_3	153	Soluble
CH_3	H	H	222	200.00
CH_3	CH_3	H	210	Soluble
CH_3	CH_3	CH_3	163	Soluble
C_6H_5	H	H	288	1.35
H	C_6H_5	H	271	2.86
CH_3	C_6H_5	H	304	0.53

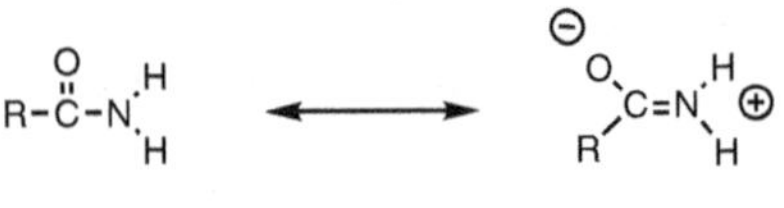

Resonance forms of amides

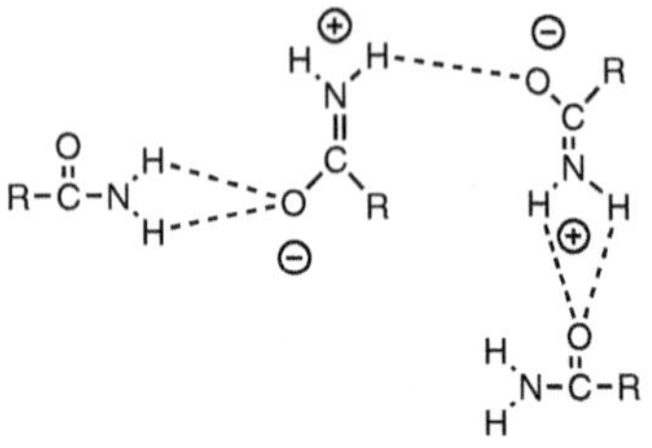

FIGURE 12-7. The effect of resonance structures of amides on intermolecular hydrogen bonding.

A chemical property that differentiates amides from esters is the greater stability of the amide. Amides are relatively stable to the acid, base, and enzymatic conditions encountered in pharmacy. The reason for this stability again can be related to the resonance forms of the amide with its overlapping clouds of electrons. The importance of the increase in stability of the amide over the ester has been used to advantage in preparing drugs with prolonged activity. Although amides are relatively stable to acid, base, and enzymes, metabolic hydrolysis can occur, catalyzed by the amidase enzymes. An example is illustrated in Figure 12-8. The important point to remember is that amides are more stable in vivo than are esters.

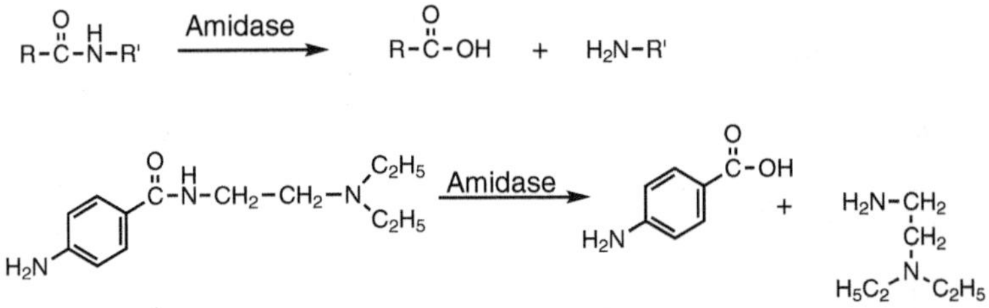

FIGURE 12-8. Metabolic hydrolysis of amides.

Although basic amines were used to prepare the amides, amides are nearly neutral functional groups, and therefore acid salts cannot be formed. Returning to the definition of a base, an unshared pair of electrons is essential for basicity. The unshared pair of electrons must be available for donation, a situation that does not exist in amides. In the amide, the pair of electrons no longer remain on the nitrogen but are spread over the nitrogen, the carbon, and the oxygen. This resonance of the electrons reduces their availability and thus the amide exhibit a neutral pH.

CARBONATES, CARBAMATES, AND UREAS

The next functional derivatives of the carboxylic acids will be grouped together because of their similarity to the previously discussed esters and amides. The carbonates, carbamates, and ureas, functional derivatives of carbonic acid, are shown below.

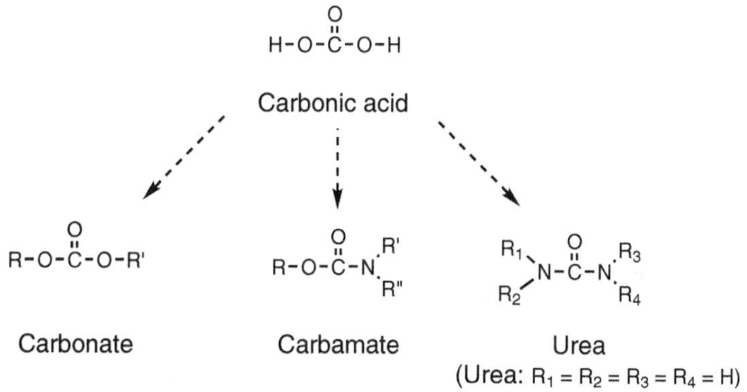

$$H-O-\overset{\overset{\displaystyle O}{\|}}{C}-O-H$$

Carbonic acid

$$R-O-\overset{\overset{\displaystyle O}{\|}}{C}-O-R'$$

Carbonate

$$R-O-\overset{\overset{\displaystyle O}{\|}}{C}-N\overset{R'}{\underset{R''}{}}$$

Carbamate

$$\overset{R_1}{\underset{R_2}{}}N-\overset{\overset{\displaystyle O}{\|}}{C}-N\overset{R_3}{\underset{R_4}{}}$$

Urea
(Urea: $R_1 = R_2 = R_3 = R_4 = H$)

■ **NOMENCLATURE.** Carbonate nomenclature may be common or official. In either case, the two alcohol portions are named and combined with the word "carbonate" (carbonates are ester derivatives of carbonic acid). An example of carbonate nomenclature is shown in Figure 12-9.

Carbamates are ester-amide derivatives of carbonic acid and, like carbonates, require the naming of the alcohol and the amine, using either common names or IUPAC nomenclature, followed by the word "carbamate" (Fig. 12-10).

The ureas, the diamide derivatives of carbonic acid, are illustrated in Figure 12-11. In this case, it may be necessary, as we see in the example, to differentiate between the two nitrogens. This is done by using N for the one nitrogen and N' for the other nitrogen. In the preceding cases, the structures should be obvious by the use of the terms "carbonate," "carbamate," and "urea" in the nomenclature.

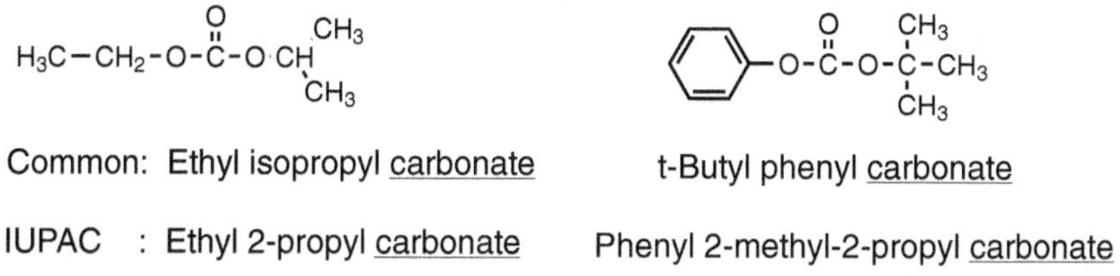

$$H_3C-CH_2-O-\overset{\overset{\displaystyle O}{\|}}{C}-O\cdot\overset{\overset{\displaystyle CH_3}{|}}{CH}\underset{CH_3}{}$$

Common: Ethyl isopropyl <u>carbonate</u>

IUPAC : Ethyl 2-propyl <u>carbonate</u>

$$\langle\!\!\langle\ \rangle\!\!\rangle-O-\overset{\overset{\displaystyle O}{\|}}{C}-O-\overset{\overset{\displaystyle CH_3}{|}}{\underset{CH_3}{C}}-CH_3$$

t-Butyl phenyl <u>carbonate</u>

Phenyl 2-methyl-2-propyl <u>carbonate</u>

FIGURE 12-9. Examples of Common and Official (IUPAC) nomenclature of carbonates.

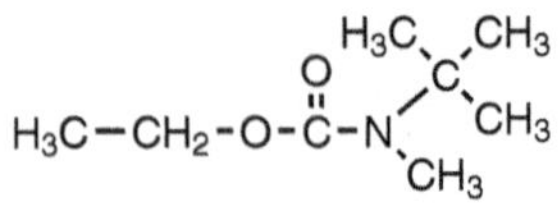

$$H_3C-CH_2-O-\overset{O}{\overset{\|}{C}}-N\overset{H_3C\,\diagdown C\diagup CH_3}{\diagdown CH_3}$$

Common: Ethyl N-methyl-N-t-butyl <u>carbamate</u>

IUPAC : Ethyl N-methyl-N-2-(2-methylpropyl) <u>carbamate</u>

FIGURE 12-10. Examples of Common and Official (IUPAC) nomenclature of carbamates.

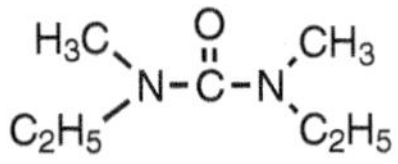

$$\underset{C_2H_5}{\overset{H_3C}{\diagdown}}N-\overset{O}{\overset{\|}{C}}-N\underset{\diagdown C_2H_5}{\overset{\diagup CH_3}{}}$$

$$\underset{C_2H_5}{\overset{C_2H_5}{\diagdown}}N-\overset{O}{\overset{\|}{C}}-N\underset{\diagdown CH_3}{\overset{\diagup CH_3}{}}$$

N,N'-Diethyl-N,N'-dimethyl <u>urea</u> 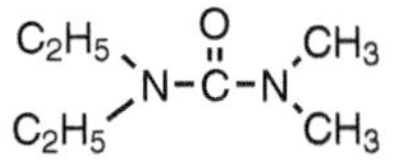   N,N-Diethyl-N',N'-dimethyl <u>urea</u>

FIGURE 12-11. Examples of nomenclature of ureas.

■ **PHYSICAL-CHEMICAL PROPERTIES.** The physical and chemical properties of the carbonate parallel those of the ester, while the properties of the urea are similar to those of the amide. The carbamate has physical properties that represent the combined effect of both components. Chemically, however, the carbamate shares reactions more like those of an ester, which means that carbonates and carbamates are unstable to acid and base conditions. The ureas, being similar to amides, are relatively nonreactive solids with the polarity properties previously discussed for amides (Fig. 12-12).

■ **METABOLISM.** The metabolic liability that these functional derivatives of carbonic acid exhibit is that of hydrolysis. This reaction is catalyzed by the esterase enzymes. Both the carbonate and the carbamate have the ester portion first hy-

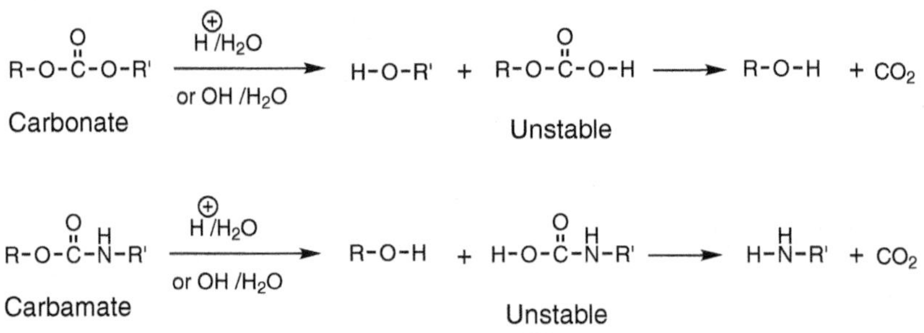

$$\underset{\text{Carbonate}}{R-O-\overset{O}{\overset{\|}{C}}-O-R'} \xrightarrow[\text{or OH}^-/H_2O]{\overset{\oplus}{H}/H_2O} H-O-R' + \underset{\text{Unstable}}{R-O-\overset{O}{\overset{\|}{C}}-O-H} \longrightarrow R-O-H + CO_2$$

$$\underset{\text{Carbamate}}{R-O-\overset{O}{\overset{\|}{C}}-\overset{H}{\underset{}{N}}-R'} \xrightarrow[\text{or OH}^-/H_2O]{\overset{\oplus}{H}/H_2O} R-O-H + \underset{\text{Unstable}}{H-O-\overset{O}{\overset{\|}{C}}-\overset{H}{\underset{}{N}}-R'} \longrightarrow H-\overset{H}{\underset{}{N}}-R' + CO_2$$

Ureas: Relatively nonreactive to aqueous acid or aqueous base

FIGURE 12-12. Acid- or base-catalyzed hydrolysis of carbonates and carbamates.

drolyzed to give the monosubstituted carbonic acid. This acid is unstable and decomposes with loss of CO_2, as shown in Figure 12-13. Carbonates are hydrolyzed with formation of carbon dioxide and alcohol, and carbamates decompose to carbon dioxide, an alcohol, and an amine. The ureas are relatively stable chemicals and are not commonly metabolized by hydrolysis.

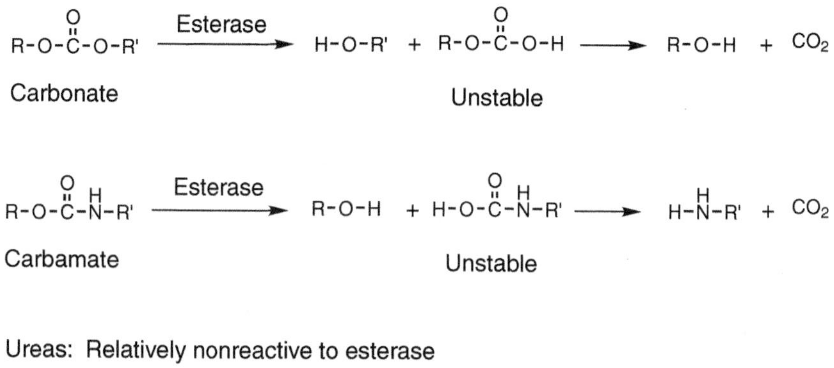

Ureas: Relatively nonreactive to esterase

FIGURE 12-13. Metabolic hydrolysis of carbonates and carbamates.

AMIDINES AND GUANIDINES

The final functional derivatives of the carboxylic acids are amidines and guanidines. Amidines are actually a functional derivative of an amide, while the guanidine is a functional derivative of urea. These two groups are mentioned since they are found as an integral part of several drug molecules. The guanidine moiety is an important unit in the naturally occurring amino acid arginine.

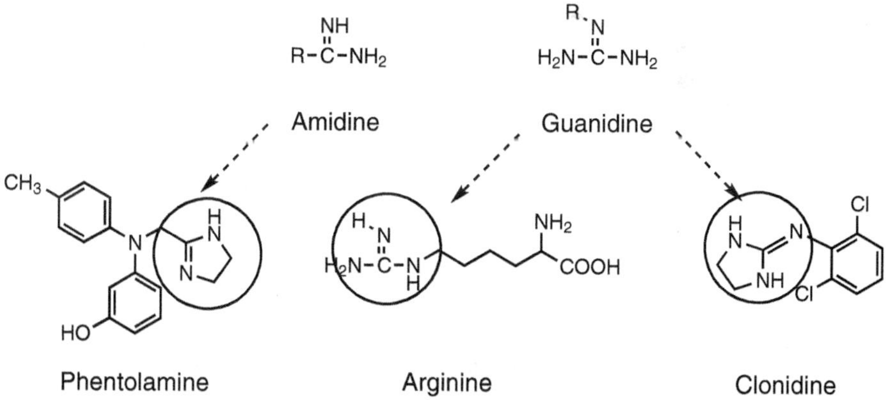

▪ **PHYSICAL-CHEMICAL PROPERTIES.** The chief characteristic of both amidines and guanidine is the high degree of basicity. In both cases the imine nitrogen maintains an unshared pair of electrons and therefore takes on a high degree of basicity. The basicity is actually increased through resonance, as indicated in

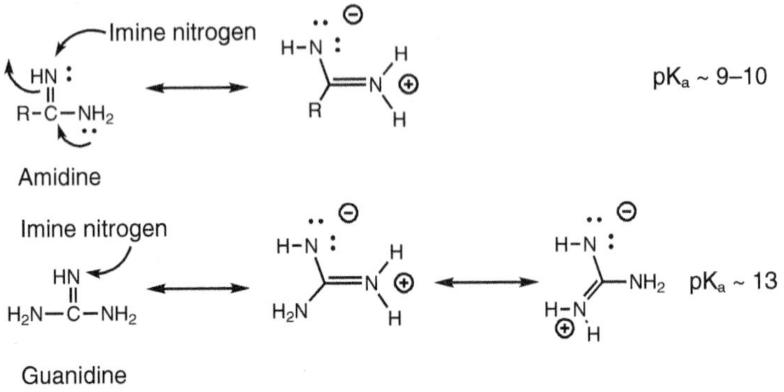

FIGURE 12-14. Basicity of amidines and guanidines.

Figure 12-14. The strength of this basicity is actually quite high. Amidines may have a pK_a of 9 to 10, while guanidines may have a pK_a as high as 13. The remaining nitrogen or nitrogens in the respective molecules remain neutral since, as indicated in Figure 12-14, the electron pair is shared by the nitrogen, the adjacent carbon, and to some extent the basic nitrogen.

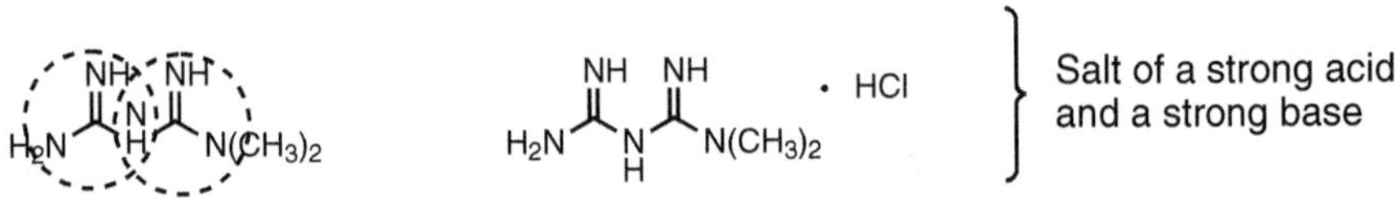

Metformin (pK_a 12.4)   Metformin hydrochloride (pK_a 6.68)
(a biguanide)

Salt of a strong acid and a strong base

Case Study 12.1

You are the chief oncology pharmacist at your community's academic medical center, and are presenting a new epothilone-based anticancer drug ixabepilone (Ixempra) to the Pharmacy and Therapeutics Committee. You tell this scientifically enlightened group of practitioners that the only structural difference between ixabepilone and the natural product epothilone B is contained within the circled component of each molecule as shown below. Ixabepilone and epothilone B act as inhibitors of cellular mitosis, a mechanism they share with the popular taxane anticancer agents paclitaxel and docetaxel.

A physician member of the Pharmacy and Therapeutics Committee is eager to probe this important chemical distinction further, and asks what therapeutic

(case study continues on page 83)

Case Study 12.1 (continued)

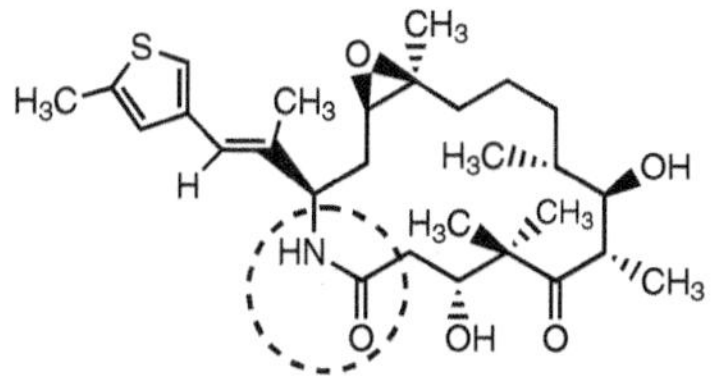

Ixabepilone (Ixempra) 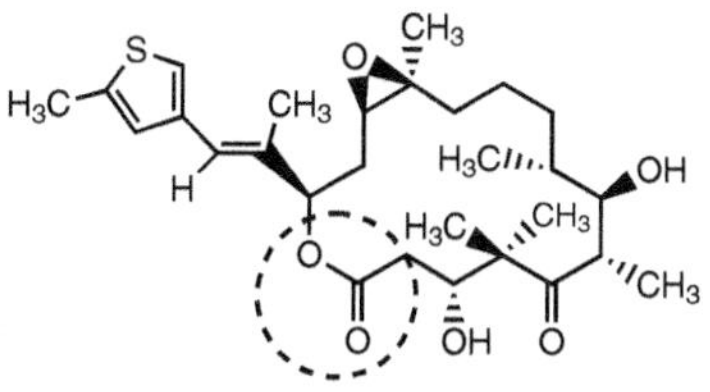   Epothilone B

advantages ixabepilone might provide over the epothilone B "parent" structure. She specifically inquires about: (1) metabolic stability, (2) in vitro stability, (3) ability to hydrogen-bond to receptor targets within the rapidly dividing cancer cell, and (4) water solubility, particularly whether ixabepilone can dissolve in water, thus avoiding the need for solubilizing agents like Cremophor EL. Cremophor EL must be used to solubilize epothilone B and paclitaxel for IV administration, and it is known to induce potentially severe hypersensitivity reactions in some patients.

Fortunately, the rock-solid knowledge of functional group chemistry you gained through your study of Lemke's Organic Functional Groups text while in pharmacy school allows you to answer this clinical question with confidence. You turn to this physician, smile, and say ....

Case Study 12.2

The year is 2020. A new acetylcholinesterase (AChE) inhibitor (psychastigmine) has been approved by the FDA for treatment of Alzheimer disease (AD). You are the pharmacist on the hospital's pharmacy and therapeutics (P&T) committee and have been asked to evaluate switching to this new drug from rivastigmine, the

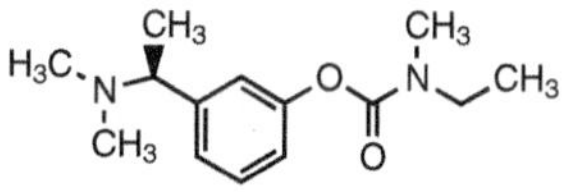

Rivastigmine 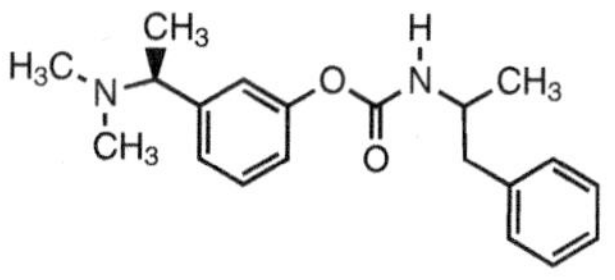   Psychastigmine

(case study continues on page 84)

Case Study 12.2 (continued)

currently approved Alzheimer treatment. You know the other members of P&T committee expect you to discuss the chemical basis of your evaluation using the chemical structure and mechanism of action.

You immediately recognize that both rivastigmine and the new psychastigmine are carbamate derivatives of carboxylic acids. They are related to an older naturally occurring carbamate AChE inhibitor, physostigmine. Physostigmine is an alkaloid isolated from the seeds of the Calabar bean (*Physostigma venenosum*) and is used mainly to treat glaucoma because its use to treat AD is limited due to its severe side effects and narrow therapeutic window. In addition you recognize the amine moiety of pyschastigmine's carbamate is a phenylethylamine that is the pharmacophore for drugs with adrenergic activity such as amphetamine.

You recall that carbamates inhibit AChE by transferring their carbamoyl group to a serine residue in the active site of AChE. The covalently bound carbamate is slowly hydrolyzed to reconstitute the active enzyme. During this process, a carbamic acid is released that in turn dissociates into carbon dioxide and an amine.

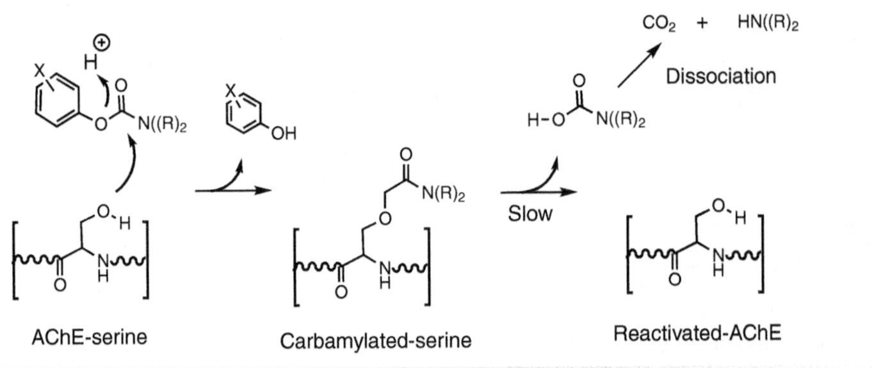

AChE-serine   Carbamylated-serine   Reactivated-AChE

With this mechanistic information and your knowledge of functional derivates of organic functional groups:

1. Would you recommend psychastigmine?
2. Explain your answer based upon the chemical reactivity and possible products.

Sulfonic Acids and Sulfonamides

Another pharmaceutically important acidic functional group is the sulfonic acid group and its amide derivatives.

SULFONIC ACIDS

■ **NOMENCLATURE.** A single nomenclature is used for sulfonic acids. This nomenclature is illustrated for several of the most common sulfonic acids (Fig. 13-1).

Pharmaceutically, the most commonly encountered sulfonic acid is methane sulfonic acid that is used to prepare water-soluble salts of basic amines. Methane sulfonates are commonly referred to as mesylates.

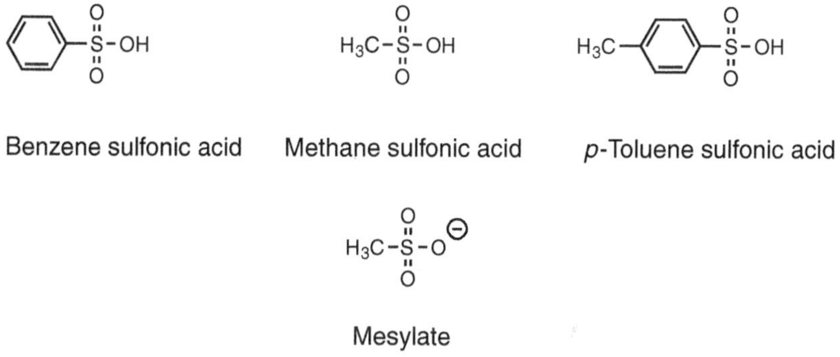

Benzene sulfonic acid   Methane sulfonic acid   *p*-Toluene sulfonic acid

Mesylate

FIGURE 13-1. Examples of nomenclature of sulfonic acids.

■ **PHYSICAL-CHEMICAL PROPERTIES.** A very significant physical-chemical property of the sulfonic acids is the pH characteristic. Sulfonic acids, in general, are strong acids, with pK_a's nearly as low as those of the mineral acids (Table 13-1). Saying that an acid is a strong acid implies that considerable dissociation occurs in water, and this suggests the possibility of ion-dipole interaction with water. By now one should know that such binding will favor water solubility. The solubility of several of these acids is shown in Table 13-1.

Table 13-1. WATER SOLUBILITY OF COMMON SULFONIC ACIDS

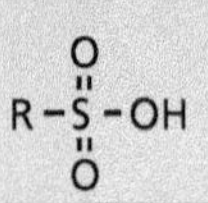 $R-\overset{\displaystyle O}{\underset{\displaystyle O}{S}}-OH$	SOLUBILITY (g/100g H_2O)	pK_a in H_2O
R = H_3C-	20.0	−1.2
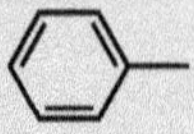 (benzene ring)	Soluble	0.7
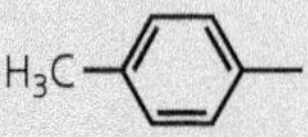 H_3C-(benzene ring)	67.0	
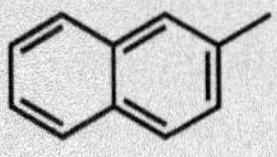 (naphthalene)	Soluble	

SULFONAMIDES

With this brief background, one now turns to the very important derivative of sulfonic acids, the sulfonamides. This group of compounds is important in medicinal chemistry, since a wide variety of drugs have the benzene sulfonamide nucleus.

■ **NOMENCLATURE.** The nomenclature for aryl sulfonamides is fairly straightforward. The name of the substituted benzene followed by the suffix "sulfonamide" is commonly used, although a few important common names will also have to be memorized, such as sulfanilamide (Fig. 13-2).

■ **PHYSICAL-CHEMICAL PROPERTIES.** The aryl sulfonamides tend to be solids with high melting points and poor water solubility. Similar to carboxylic acid amides, aryl sulfonamides are chemically quite stable. Benzene sulfonamides are stable to acid, base, and enzymatic hydrolysis.

Unlike the carboxylic acid amides, which are considered neutral compounds, the aryl sulfonamides are weak acids. The acidic nature results from the ability of the SO_2 moiety to stabilize the nitrogen anion through resonance (Fig. 13-3). In the presence of a strong base, such as sodium or potassium hydroxide, aryl sulfonamides will react to form a salt (Fig. 13-4). The sodium or potassium salt of a sulfonamide will readily dissociate in water, leading to highly water-soluble products, the result of ion-dipole bonding. The pH of the aqueous media following dissolution of a sodium or potassium salt of a sulfonamide tends to be quite alkaline. The water-soluble salts of aryl sulfonamides are incompatible with acidic media since an acid-base reaction can occur, usually leading to precipitation of the aryl sulfonamide.

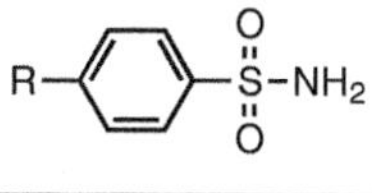

R	Common name	IUPAC name
H-	Benzene sulfonamide	Benzene sulfonamide
H_3C-	p-Toluene sulfonamide	4-Methylbenzene sulfonamide
H_2N-	p-Aminobenzene sulfonamide Sulfanilamide	4-Aminobenzene sulfonamide

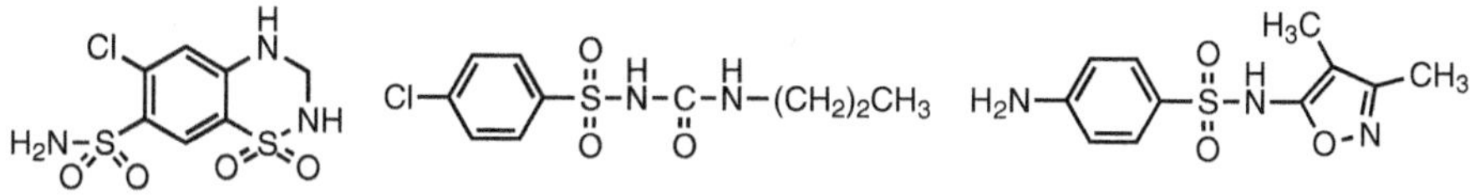

Hydrochlorothiazide   Chlorpropamide   Sulfisoxazole

FIGURE 13-2. Aryl sulfonamides nomenclature and drug examples.

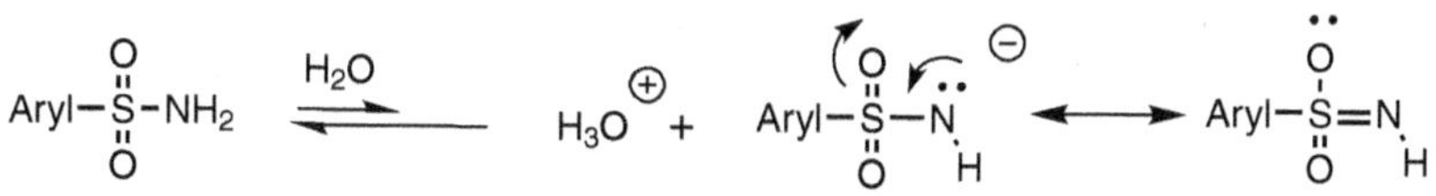

FIGURE 13-3. Acidity of sulfonamides.

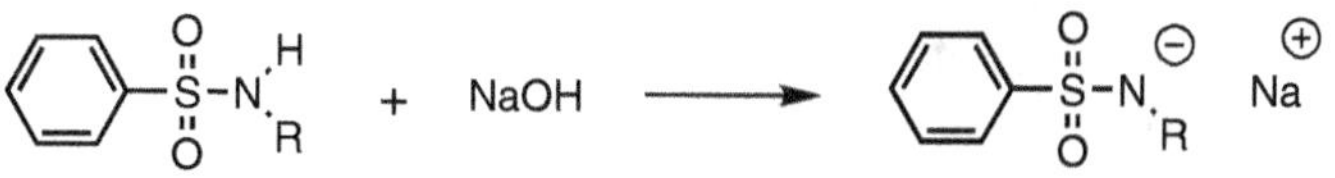

Water-soluble

FIGURE 13-4. Salt formation of benzene sulfonamide.

Case Study 13.1

You are returning for a third year to a summer job at a generic pharmaceutical company conveniently located in your hometown. Having had the wisdom to take several organic chemistry-focused elective courses during your prepharmacy and pharmacy program, you supervise the activity of several technicians in a laboratory focused on sulfonamide-containing drugs.

(case study continues on page 88)

Case Study 13.1 (continued)

A newly hired tech has approached you to report a problem he's having in synthesizing the sodium salt of one of the company's products. He had no trouble with the other two compounds he was working on, but he just can't get the third to generate the water-soluble salt he anticipated. He shows you the structure of the three drugs on his bench.

1. Which of the three sulfonamides was giving this new technician such a difficult time, and why?
2. Would you advise this technician to try to make the hydrochloride salt (e.g., by reacting the recalcitrant structure with HCl rather than NaOH)? Why or why not?

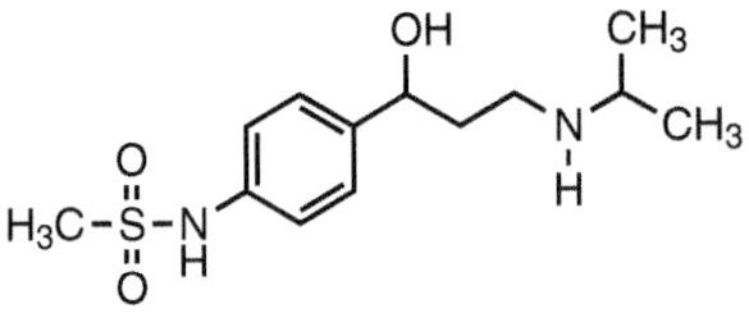

1

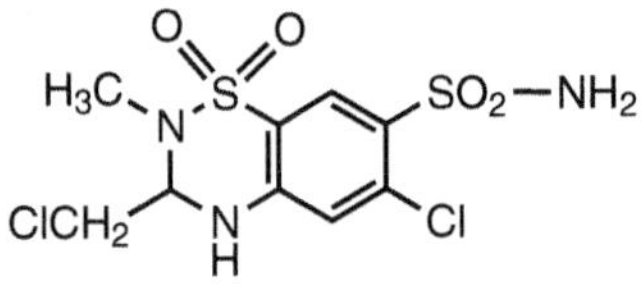

3

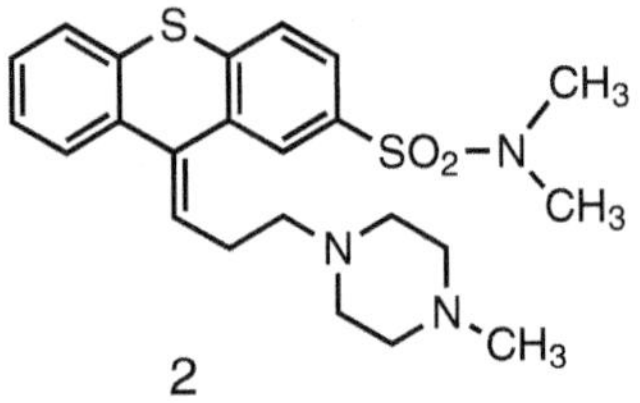

2

Case Study 13.2

Your uncle is a physician. He relates to you a case he recently had in treating an HIV-positive patient with sulfadiazine (5 g/day) and pyrimethamine (100 mg/day) for

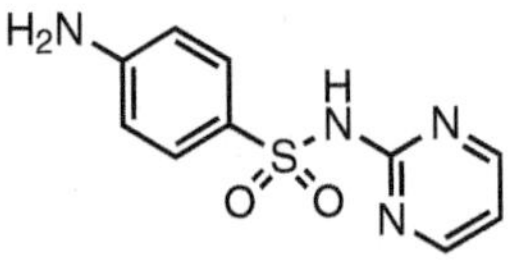

Sulfadiazine

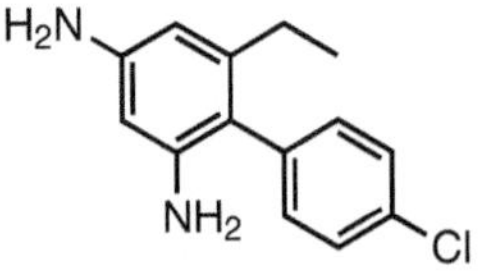

Pyrimethamine

(case study continues on page 89)

Case Study 13.2 (continued)

toxoplasmic encephalitis, the treatment of choice. After several days of therapy the patient developed hematuria and mild renal failure (serum creatinine 130 μmol/L). The patient's urinary pH was 6.0 and the urine sediment of the patient showed crystals that were identified as sulfadiazine (pK$_a$ = 6.5) and its N^4-acetylsulfadiazine metabolite (pK$_a$ = 6.4).

Knowing that you are a P-1 student your uncle tests your knowledge by asking you if you can explain:

1. Why sulfadiazine formed crystals in this patient's kidneys?
2. What physicochemical recommendation would you make to correct this condition?

You recall from a previous discussion of amines that aromatic amines can undergo phase 2 metabolic conjugation with glucuronic acid, sulfuric acid, and/or acetyl coenzyme A while sulfonamides do not undergo any commonly identified metabolism.

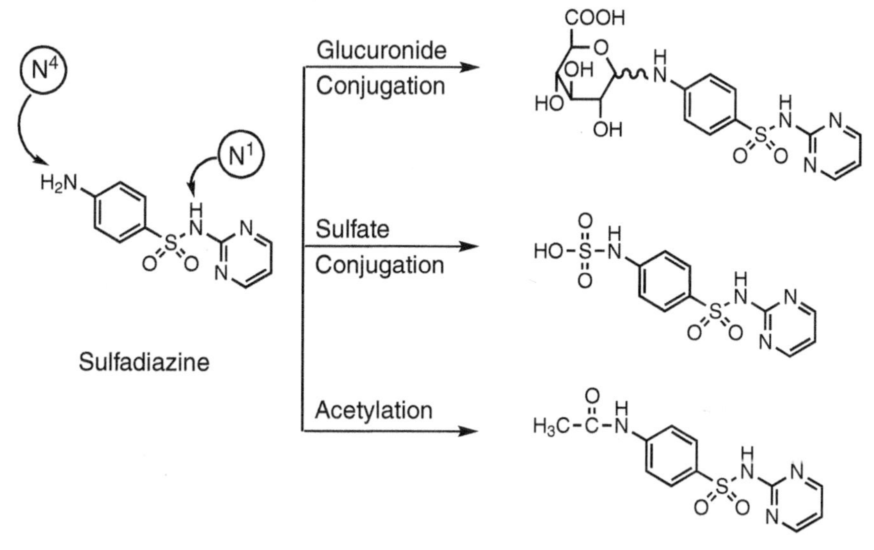

Nitrogen Functional Groups

14

NITRO GROUPS

A common functional group found in many drug molecules is the organic bound nitro group. In most cases the nitro is present as an aromatic bound nitro such as those shown in Figure 14-1. While official nomenclature for drug molecules containing the nitro may be quite complicated, one should recognize the presence of a nitro group since this group is named as "nitro" in the official nomenclature. Although the nitro group is a neutral functional group, the resonance structures of this group exhibit charged species, as shown, and account for the strong electron withdrawing properties of the group.

Metabolism of aryl nitro groups is that of reduction to the arylamine (see Fig. 14-2). The reduction intermediates, one of which is the hydroxylamine, have been implicated as possible carcinogens.

NITRATE GROUP

Among the cardiac agents one finds a group of drugs known as the organic nitrates. One of the better known drugs in this class is nitroglycerin (Fig. 14-3), which is

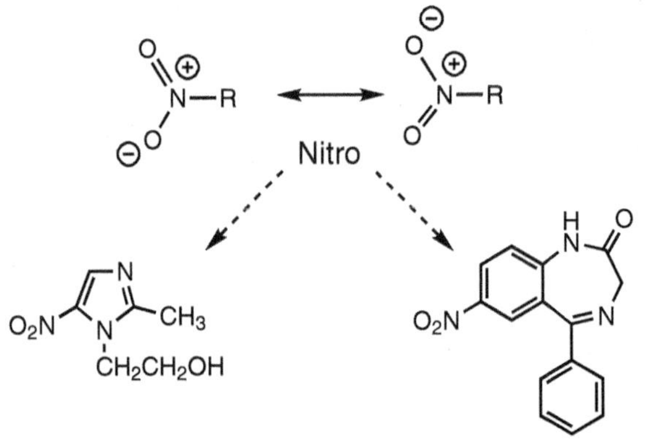

Metronidazole
(2-Methyl-5-**nitro**imidazole-
1-ethanol)

Nitrazapam
(1,3-Dihydro-7-**nitro**-5-phenyl-
2H-1,4-benzodiazepine-2-one)

FIGURE 14-1. Examples of the nitro group in drug molecules.

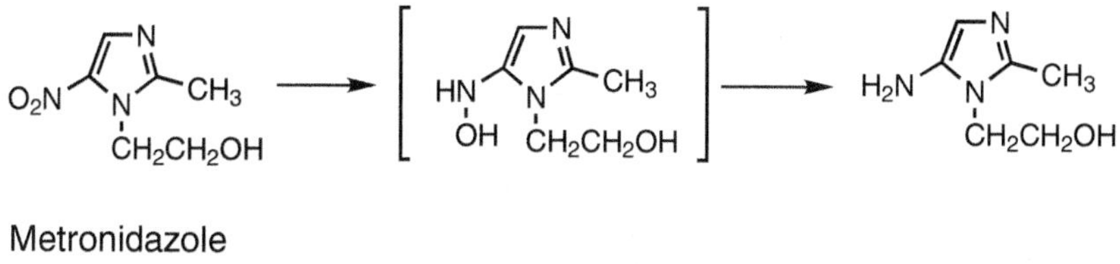

Metronidazole

FIGURE 14-2. Metabolism of the arylnitro group.

actually an ester of nitric acid plus the triol glycerin. The nitrate ester structure accounts for a potential instability in that simple hydrolysis can lead to formation of nitric acid and the free alcohol. This reaction can also occur in vivo and represents a potential metabolic fate.

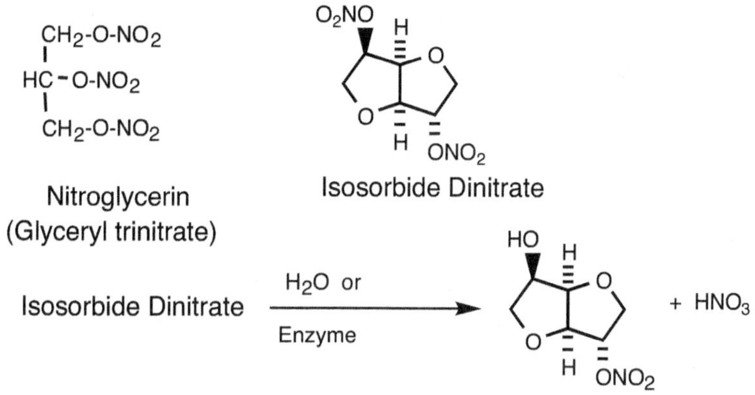

CH_2-O-NO_2
|
HC-O-NO_2
|
CH_2-O-NO_2

Nitroglycerin
(Glyceryl trinitrate)

Isosorbide Dinitrate

Isosorbide Dinitrate $\xrightarrow{\text{H}_2\text{O or Enzyme}}$ + HNO_3

FIGURE 14-3. Organic nitrates and their potential hydrolysis.

NITRITE GROUP

Although not common, the nitrite functional group appears in the drug amyl nitrite and consists of an ester of nitrous acid and amyl alcohol. The nitrates and amyl nitrite appear to produce their beneficial effects by releasing NO.

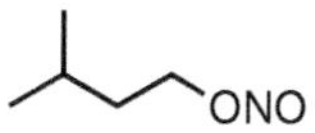

Amyl nitrite

OXIMES

The oxime functional group has found significant application in a number of drug classes, but especially in the cephalosporin class of antibiotics. Formed from the reaction of a ketone or aldehyde with hydroxylamine, two geometrical isomers may form (Fig. 14-4). Based upon specific priority rules, when the highest priority substituent (R or R′) and the OH group are on the same side of the double bond this is given the *Z* designation (or *syn* configuration) and when the highest priority substituent (R or R′) and the OH group are on the opposite side of the double bond this is given the *E* designation (or *anti* configuration). The resulting oxime is generally considered neutral.

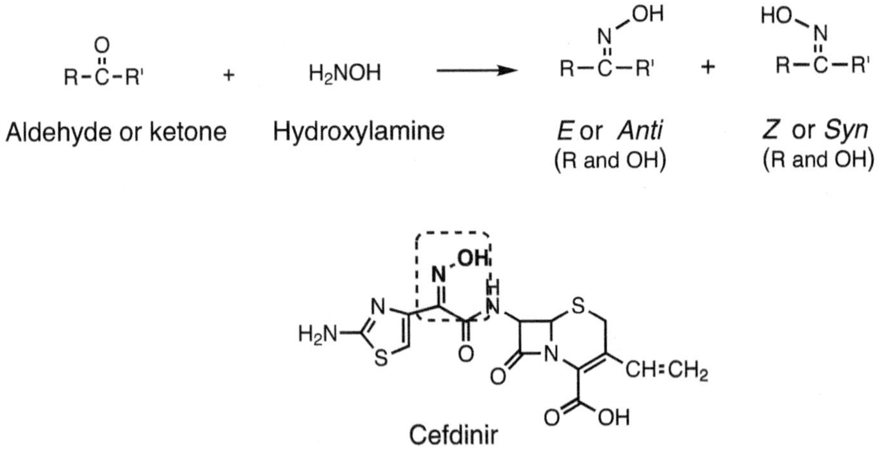

FIGURE 14-4. Formation of oximes from ketones or aldehydes.

HYDRAZONE/HYDRAZINE/HYDRAZIDE

Similar to the oxime, the reaction of an aldehyde or ketone with hydrazine gives rise to a hydrazone (Fig. 14-5). The formation of a carbon–nitrogen double bond is referred to as a Schiff base, while this functionality is known as an imine. Schiff base formation occurs commonly in biochemical systems when a primary amine reacts with a ketone or aldehyde. The resulting hydrazone is unstable to aqueous acid and will hydrolyze back to hydrazine and the ketone or aldehyde. Both the imine nitrogen and the −NH₂ nitrogen in the hydrazone are basic. As with oximes, hydrazones can exist as geometric isomers, but there are no drug examples where separation of the isomers has been reported. Reduction of the hydrazone leads to formation of the hydrazine. The hydrazine is stable to acid or base hydrolysis and has basic properties. Finally, acetylation of one of the nitrogens gives rise to a hydrazide in which the −NH₂ nitrogen retains its basic properties while the −NH nitrogen acts like a neutral amide.

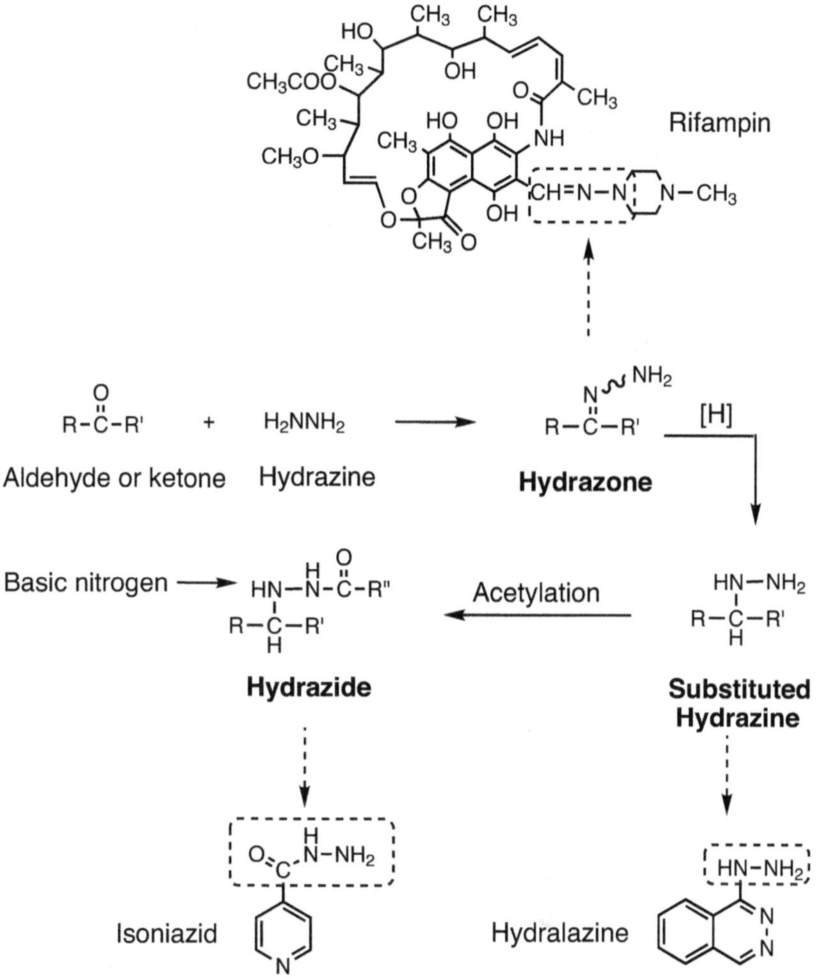

FIGURE 14-5. Hydrazine derivatives and drug examples.

Case Study 14.1

As president of your pharmacy school's student body, you have worked hard with your counterparts in your state's 10 other pharmacy programs to organize the first *"Use It Or Lose It"* drug chemistry knowledge competition. Medicinal chemists and clinical pharmacy faculty from all programs are serving as the panel of examiners, and they have jointly developed questions that emphasize the essential role of chemistry in predicting drug action.

(case study continues on page 94)

Case Study 14.1 (continued)

Your school is currently tied for first place with the team from top seed Wyknott U., and you are representing your team in the final round of the competition. Wyknott just blew a tough question on nitrogen functional groups, and the pressure is on. If you answer the question correctly, your school will win the competition, and big scholarship bucks will be awarded to everyone on your team.

Are you ready to be the hero? Then just answer the following question:

> H_2 antagonists decrease the risk of gastrointestinal ulceration and heartburn by blocking histamine-induced gastric acid secretion. Some H_2 antagonists contain a diaminoethene group that must be substituted with a polar, electron withdrawing functional group (R). If a net positive charge is allowed to form in this molecular area, the pharmacological activity changes from H_2 antagonist (ulcer-preventing) to H_2 agonist (ulcer-promoting). Given the above, which of the following nitrogen-containing functional groups have the properties needed to retain H_2 antagonist activity if used for the "R" substituent on diaminoethene-based H_2 antagonists?

Diaminoethene

R = polar, electron withdrawing, noncationic

H_2 Antagonist

1. $-NO_2$

2. $-CH=N-OH$

3. $-CH=N-NH_2$

4. $-C-\overset{H}{\underset{\parallel}{N}}-NH_2$, with $\parallel$ O

Case Study 14.2

You are a first year pharmacy student. You chose pharmacy as a profession because of your interest in chemistry which was developed in you by your high school chemistry teacher. You want to pursue your interest in chemistry by volunteering to work in your medicinal chemistry teacher's laboratory. The professor smiles at you and welcomes your enthusiasm; however, he tells you that he has been disappointed by students in the past so before he accepts your proposal he challenges you to evaluate what you see in the following three drug structures. He says he knows you have only had the organic functional group course and only expects you to evaluate the circled

(case study continues on page 95)

Case Study 14.2 (continued)

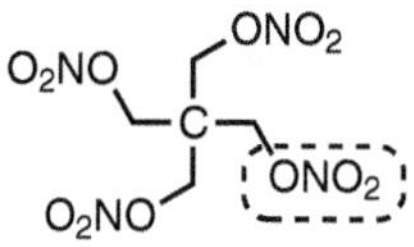

Pentaerythritol tetranitrate

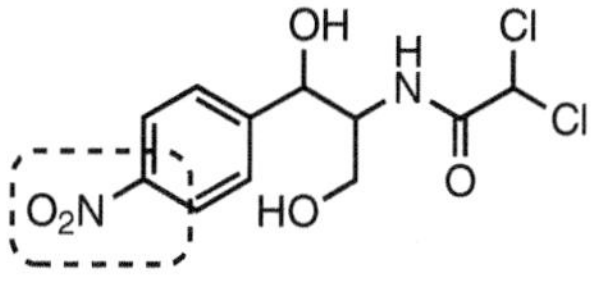

Chloramphenicol

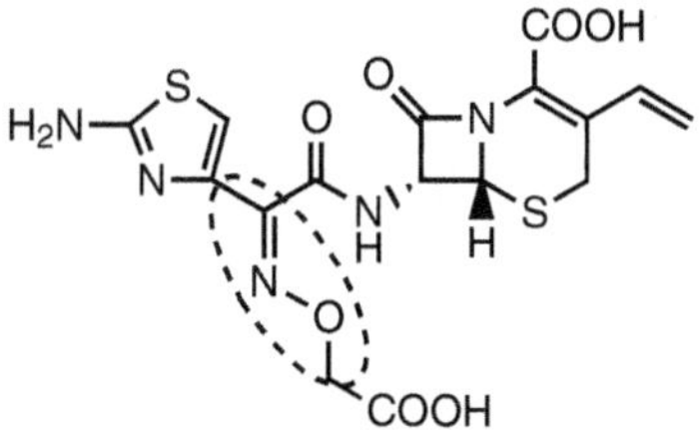

Cefixime

functional groups. He considers the ability to look at a chemical structure and "read" what its functional groups "tell" you as a key indication of a student's ability in the chemistry laboratory. The professor hands you a piece of chalk and sends you to the blackboard.

Heterocycles

15

This chapter introduces the subject of heterocyclic chemistry. *Heterocycles* are defined as cyclic molecules that contain one or more heteroatoms in a ring. A *heteroatom* is an atom other than carbon. One need merely glance through an index of biologically active structures to recognize the array of heterocycles found in synthetic and naturally occurring molecules. A background in heterocyclic chemistry is therefore highly desirable. The competencies expected of you from this section of the book consist of:

1. The ability to match a structure of a heterocycle to its common or official name
2. The ability to list the physical and chemical properties of representative heterocycles
3. The ability to draw the structure of expected metabolites of common heterocycles

It would be impossible to introduce all of the possible heterocycles that are of medicinal value within the limitations of this book. I have selected a limited number of monocyclic, bicyclic, and tricyclic rings and will confine the discussion to the heteroatoms of oxygen, nitrogen, and sulfur. In addition, only three-, four-, five-, six-, seven-, and eight-membered monocyclic heterocycles will be considered, along with the five-six, six-six, and six-seven bicyclic heterocycles. Several important tricyclic rings will also be considered. In systematic nomenclature, one will recognize a consistent form of nomenclature that follows certain rules for naming the heteroatom and ring size. Tables 15-1 and 15-2 list the rules for heterocyclic systems. In addition, as will be noted in the nomenclature section for the individual heterocycles, the numbering of heterocycles usually begins with the heteroatom being designated as the 1 position. In heterocycles that contain multiple heteroatoms, the convention is that in numbering, the oxygen atom has priority over the sulfur atom, which in turn has priority over the nitrogen atom.

THREE-MEMBERED RING HETEROCYCLES

Oxygen

■ **NOMENCLATURE.** A saturated three-membered ring containing oxygen is known as the oxirane (Fig. 15-1) ring according to the rules presented in Tables 15-1 and 15-2. While correctly named as oxiranes, the common practice for such molecules is to refer to these agents as epoxides. A number of natural products can be found

Table 15-1. ACCEPTABLE PREFIXES FOR COMMON HETEROATOMS

ELEMENT	PREFIX
Oxygen	Oxa
Nitrogen	Aza
Sulfur	Thia

Table 15-2. COMMON SUFFIXES FOR NITROGEN-CONTAINING HETEROCYCLES AND NON-NITROGEN-CONTAINING HETEROCYCLES BASED ON RING SIZE

RING SIZE	SATURATED	PARTLY SATURATED	UNSATURATED
		Rings with Nitrogen	
3	-iridine		-irine
5	-olidine	-oline	-ole
6	-ine	(di or tetrahydro)	-ine
7	(hexahydro)	(di or tetrahydro)	-epine
8	(octahydro)	(di, tetra, or hexahydro)	-ocine
		Rings without Nitrogen	
3	-irane		-irene
5	-olane	-olene	-ole
6	-ane	(di or tetrahydro)	-ine
7	-epane	(di or tetrahydro)	-epine
8	-ocane	(di, tetra, or hexahydro)	-ocin

that contain the epoxide functional group, and you will be introduced to additional epoxide-containing drugs in medicinal chemistry.

■ **PHYSICAL-CHEMICAL PROPERTIES.** Epoxides are ethers, but because of the three-membered ring, epoxides have unusual properties. The three-membered ring forces the atoms making up the ring to have an average bond angle of 60°, considerably less than the normal tetrahedral bond angle of 109.5°. This highly strained ring therefore readily opens in the presence of either acid or base catalysts, as shown in Figure 15-2. These reactions are important, since drugs that contain an epoxide ring are also quite reactive both in vitro and in vivo. Such drugs will

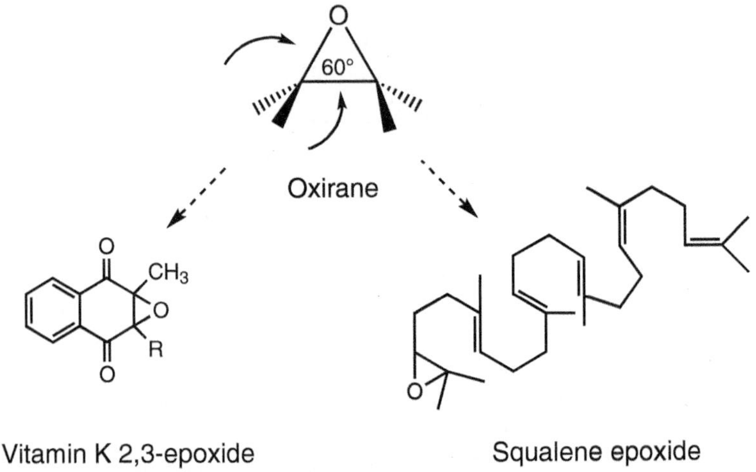

Vitamin K 2,3-epoxide   Squalene epoxide

FIGURE 15-1. Oxirane and examples of natural occurring oxiranes.

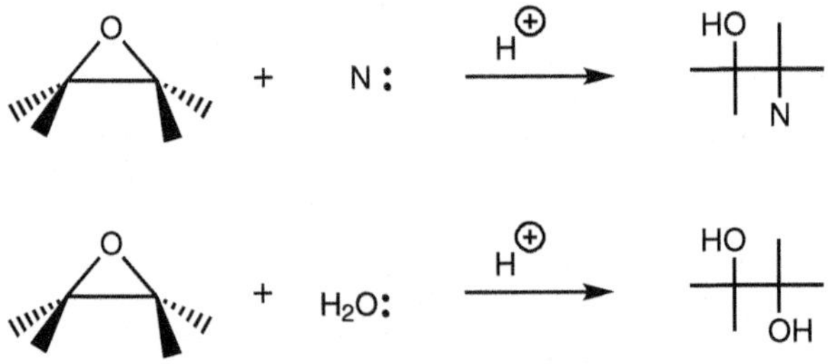

FIGURE 15-2. Acid- or base-catalyzed ring opening reactions of epoxides.

react with a nucleophile (N:) in the presence of acid or will react with a base that acts as a nucleophile to give open-chain compounds. When drugs containing epoxides are administered to a patient, the epoxide can be expected to react with biopolymers (e.g., proteins), leading to destructive effects on the cell. Such drugs may find use in cancer chemotherapy but are usually found to be quite toxic.

Nitrogen

■ **NOMENCLATURE.** A saturated three-membered ring containing nitrogen is known as the aziridine ring (Fig. 15-3). This is the only nomenclature used for such a unit. Although aziridine rings are not common in nature or in many drugs, their intermediacy is required and accounts for the biologic activity of a specific class of anticancer drugs known as the nitrogen mustards.

■ **PHYSICAL-CHEMICAL PROPERTIES.** Similar to the properties of the epoxide, aziridines are highly strained, highly reactive molecules. The anticancer drug

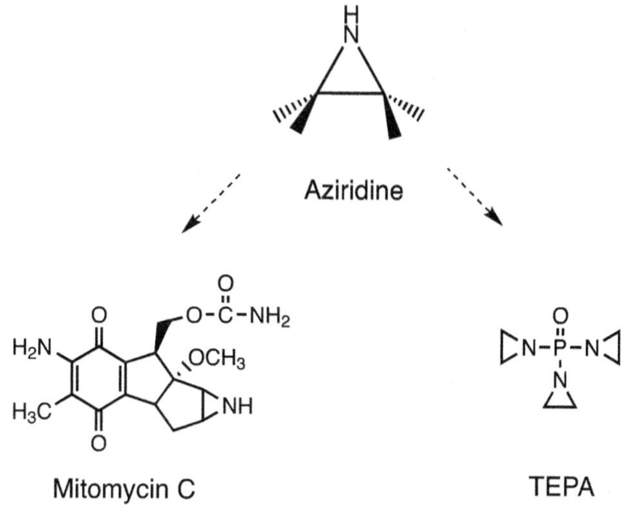

Aziridine

O-C-NH₂

H₂N

OCH₃

H₃C

NH

O

Mitomycin C

O
N-P-N
N

TEPA

FIGURE 15-3. Aziridine and examples of drugs containing aziridines.

mechlorethamine (Fig. 15-4) owes its activity to the formation of a charged intermediate aziridine (aziridinium ion). Because of its high reactivity, aziridine will react with most nucleophiles (N:), including water. If the nucleophile is part of a biopolymer, this reaction, known as an alkylation reaction, can result in the death of the cell. This reaction is either beneficial, where the cell is a cancer cell, or the mechanism of toxicity, where the cell is a host cell. The drug mechlorethamine has only a short half-life when dissolved in water because the aziridinium ion, when formed, reacts with water to give an alcohol that does not possess biologic activity.

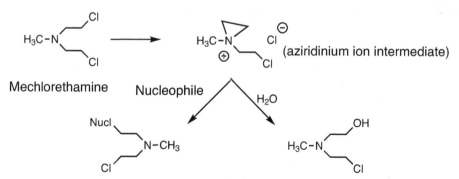

FIGURE 15-4. Aziridine as a reactive intermediate formed from mechlorethamine.

FOUR-MEMBERED RING HETEROCYCLES

Only one derivative of a four-membered ring heterocycle will be mentioned here. This system is the β-lactam, a unit found in the penicillin and cephalosporin

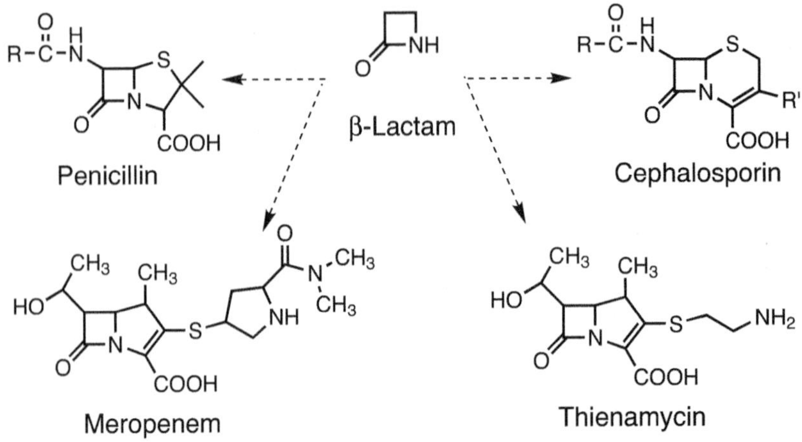

FIGURE 15-5. β-Lactam and examples of drugs containing the β-lactam.

antibiotics as well as a number of derivatives, both synthetic and naturally occurring, of these well-known antibiotics (Fig. 15-5). The nomenclature for this heterocycle is derived from the fact that cyclic amides are known as lactams, and this particular system results from cyclization of a β-aminocarboxylic acid, thus the β-lactam name. The notable property of the β-lactam, its ease of hydrolysis by aqueous acid, aqueous base, and enzymatic conditions, results from the considerable strain energy found in this molecule. The four-membered ring distorts the normal bond angles for carbon, but additionally the presence of the sp^2 carbonyl carbon adds to this strain. The hydrolysis of the β-lactam (Fig. 15-6) is a significant problem experienced by many of the penicillins, cephalosporins, and other β-lactam-containing antibiotics.

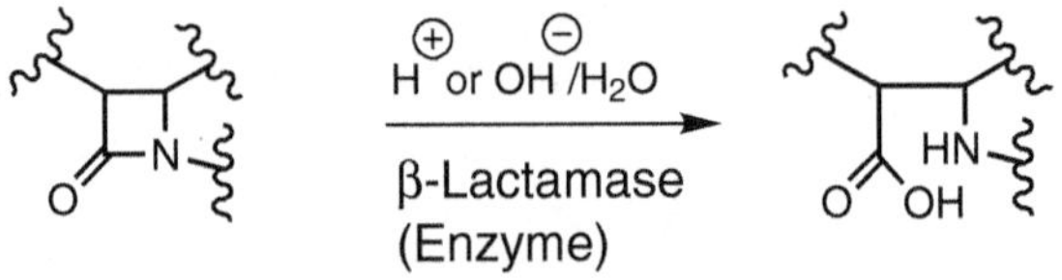

FIGURE 15-6. Hydrolysis of β-lactams.

FIVE-MEMBERED RING HETEROCYCLES

Oxygen

■ **NOMENCLATURE.** Two common five-membered ring heterocycles are furan and tetrahydrofuran (Fig. 15-7). With this ring system, you need not be concerned with official nomenclature; the common or trivial name will be used in nearly all cases. Substituted furans and tetrahydrofurans are numbered starting with the

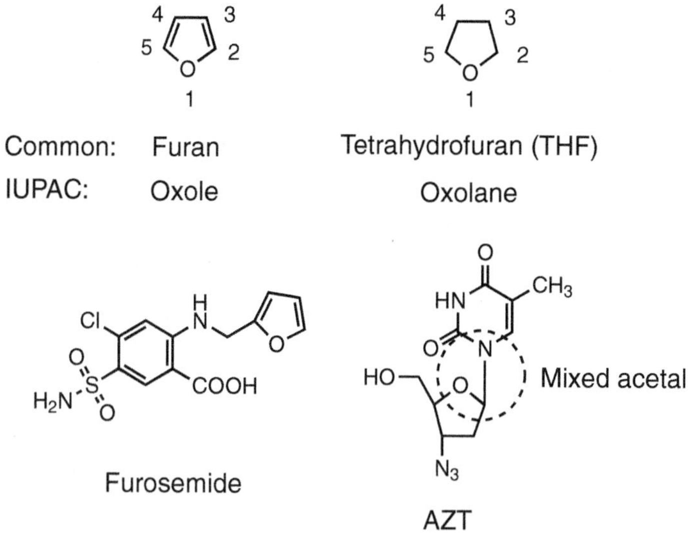

FIGURE 15-7. Five-membered oxygen containing heterocycles and examples of drugs containing these rings.

oxygen as the 1 position and numbering the ring such that any substituents receive the next lowest number.

A number of furan-containing drugs can be found, while virtually no pure tetrahydrofuran-containing drugs exist. What appears to be a tetrahydrofuran is seen in the ribose-containing anticancer and antiviral drugs, but these sugars are actually mixed acetal structures.

■ **PHYSICAL-CHEMICAL PROPERTIES.** Although furan looks like an ether, it does not behave like one; its properties are more like those of benzene. Furan is an aromatic ring. You may recall that aromatic rings are flat molecules that contain $4N + 2\pi$ electrons, in which $N = 1, 2, 3$, etc. If one considers the π electrons or sp^2 electrons present in furan, it will be noted that furan contains four π electrons in the two double bonds and two pairs of sp^2 electrons on the oxygen. One pair of the electrons on oxygen is in the same plane with the four π electrons of the two double bonds, thus resulting in a cloud of six electrons located above and below the plane of the ring (Fig. 15-8). Furan therefore has the properties of an aromatic compound: namely, it is relatively nonreactive under the conditions encountered in pharmacy. On the other hand, tetrahydrofuran has quite different properties when compared to furan. Tetrahydrofuran is simply a cyclic ether but unlike its closest open-chain relative, diethylether, does not show partial water solubility; it is highly soluble in water. This is due to the strong bonding between the hydrogen of water and the unshared pairs of electrons on the ether oxygen (Fig. 15-9).

Tetrahydrofuran is easily oxidized in the presence of air to give peroxides and, like most ethers, also must be protected from atmospheric oxygen.

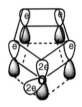

FIGURE 15-8. π Electron structure of furan.

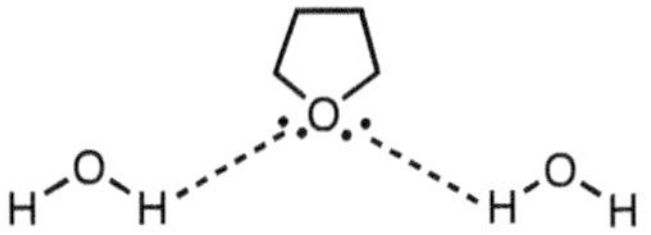

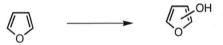

FIGURE 15-9. Strong dipole-dipole bonding in THF leading to increased water solubility.

■ **METABOLISM.** The metabolism of furan and tetrahydrofuran follow the pattern expected for an aromatic compound and an ether, respectively. While tetrahydrofuran is relatively stable in vivo, furan may undergo the expected aromatic hydroxylation (Fig. 15-10).

FIGURE 15-10. Metabolic hydroxylation of furan.

Nitrogen

■ **NOMENCLATURE.** Two common five-membered ring heterocycles containing nitrogen are pyrrole and pyrrolidine (Fig. 15-11). Here again, the common name should be learned; the official name can be neglected since it is seldom used. For substituted pyrroles or pyrrolidines, the numbering starts with nitrogen and proceeds clockwise or counterclockwise to give any substituent present the next lowest number. The pyrrole and pyrrolidine heterocycles are common features in many drugs and naturally occurring substances.

■ **PHYSICAL-CHEMICAL PROPERTIES.** Pyrrole, like furan, is an aromatic compound. It is an aromatic compound that is a weak base and, for our purposes, will be considered neutral. This property can be explained by accounting for all of the nonbonding electrons present in pyrrole (Fig. 15-12). Nitrogen's extra pair of electrons,

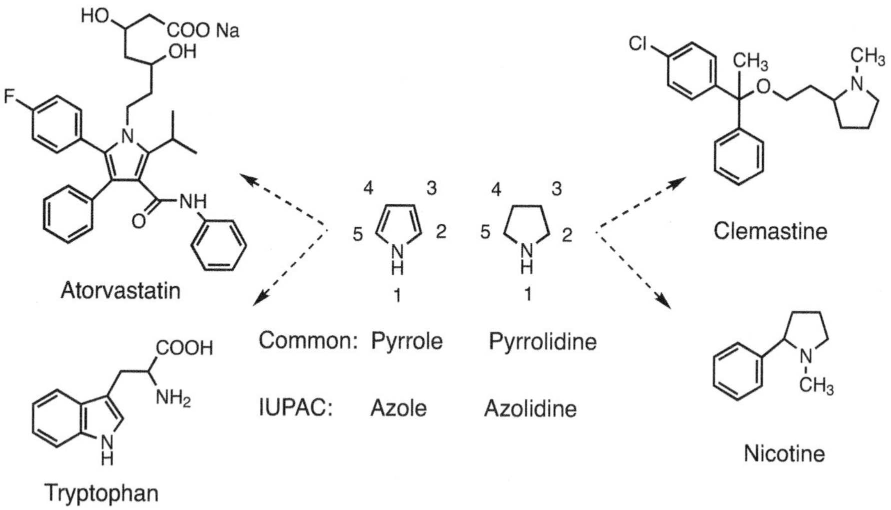

Atorvastatin

Tryptophan

Common:	Pyrrole	Pyrrolidine
IUPAC:	Azole	Azolidine

Clemastine

Nicotine

FIGURE 15-11. Pyrrole and pyrrolidine and examples of drugs containing these heterocycles.

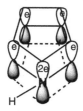

FIGURE 15-12. π Electron structure of pyrrole.

which are usually available for sharing and account for the basic properties of amines, are not available for sharing. This pair of electrons is part of the π cloud of electrons.

In the fully reduced heterocycle, pyrrolidine, one is dealing with a secondary amine with properties equivalent to any other secondary amine. Unlike pyrrole, with a pK_a of the protonated pyrrole of approximately 0.4, pyrrolidine is a strong base, with a pK_a of the ammonium ion of approximately 11. As might be expected, pyrrolidine, with only four carbon atoms and the availability of an unshared pair of electrons for hydrogen bonding, is quite water-soluble.

▪ **METABOLISM.** The metabolism of pyrrole and pyrrolidine, as well as of pyrrole- and pyrrolidine-containing molecules, follows the pattern expected for an aromatic compound and a secondary amine, respectively. Aromatic hydroxylation would be predicted for pyrrole, while pyrrolidine could be expected to undergo conjugation with glucuronic acid or sulfuric acid. Acetylation, a common reaction for secondary amines, might also be expected to occur (see Fig. 10-10, page 57).

Sulfur

■ **NOMENCLATURE.** As with the previous oxygen and nitrogen heterocycles, two sulfur-containing heterocycles, thiophene and tetrahydrothiophene, exist. Here again, the common nomenclature is used in most instances. With substituted analogs, the numbering of the rings starts with the heteroatom, proceeding either clockwise or counterclockwise, such that any substituent receives the next lowest number (Fig. 15-13). While the thiophene nucleus is common in drug molecules, the tetrahydrothiophene is quite uncommon.

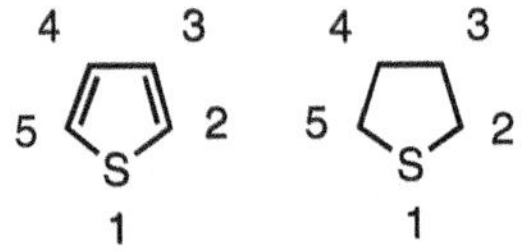

Common: Thiophene   Tetrahydrothiophene

IUPAC: Thiole   Thiolane

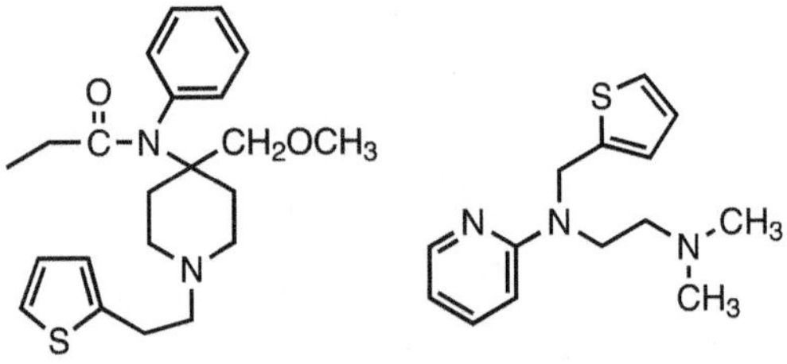

Sufentanil   Methapyrilene

FIGURE 15-13. Thiophene and tetrahydrothiophene and examples of drugs containing the thiophene heterocycle.

■ **PHYSICAL-CHEMICAL PROPERTIES.** The properties of the five-membered sulfur-containing heterocycles are based upon the proper recognition of the class of compounds to which they belong. Thiophene is an aromatic ring and is therefore relatively stable, while tetrahydrothiophene is a thioether. Unlike oxygen ethers, the thioethers are fairly stable compounds and, also unlike the oxygen analogs, the sulfur-containing compounds are less water-soluble. In general, the substitution of sulfur for oxygen results in a significant decrease in hydrophilic character and a corresponding increase in lipophilic character.

■ **METABOLISM.** The predicted metabolic pattern for thiophene is aromatic hydroxylation, with hydroxylation occurring at any hydrogen-substituted position. For reduced thiophenes, tetrahydrothiophene, oxidation of sulfur would be predicted to occur. This was previously discussed for thioethers and is again shown in Figure 15-14.

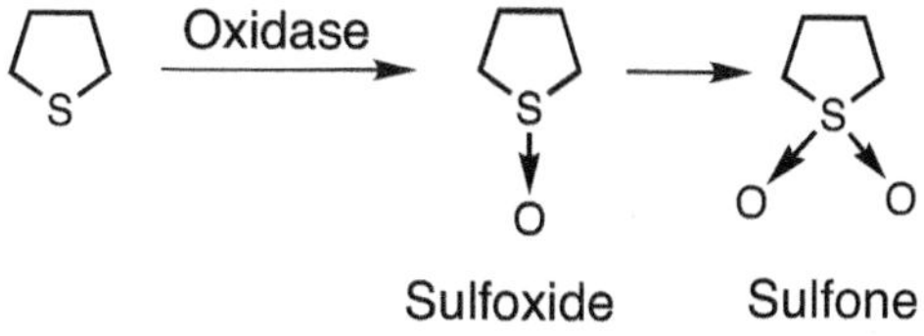

Sulfoxide   Sulfone

FIGURE 15-14. Metabolic oxidation of tetrahydrothiophene.

FIVE-MEMBERED RING HETEROCYCLES WITH TWO OR MORE HETEROATOMS

Oxygen and Nitrogen

■ **NOMENCLATURE.** Oxygen-plus-nitrogen in a five-membered ring gives rise to the heterocycles oxazole and isoxazole. The oxazole nomenclature is similar to its official name, but for convenience the -1,3- is dropped, and it is understood that oxazole consists of the 1,3 arrangement of oxygen and nitrogen. The only other arrangement of these two atoms in a five-membered ring would be the 1,2 placement. Since this is an isomer of oxazole, the common name is isoxazole (Fig. 15-15). As indicated previously, the numbering of the ring proceeds from oxygen at the 1 position to nitrogen such that the nitrogen is the next lowest position (i.e., 3 in oxazole or 2 in isoxazole).

The partially and totally reduced derivatives of oxazole are also shown. The nomenclature is based upon the general rules presented in Table 15-2. Depending on the substitution at the 2 position, oxazolidine is actually a mixed acetal (R = H, alkyl or aryl; R′ = H) or a mixed ketal (R = alkyl, aryl; R′ = alkyl or aryl) (see page 45).

On several occasions reference has been made to mixed acetals or mixed ketals (Fig. 10-11 and corresponding discussion). Oxazolidine is an example of a mixed

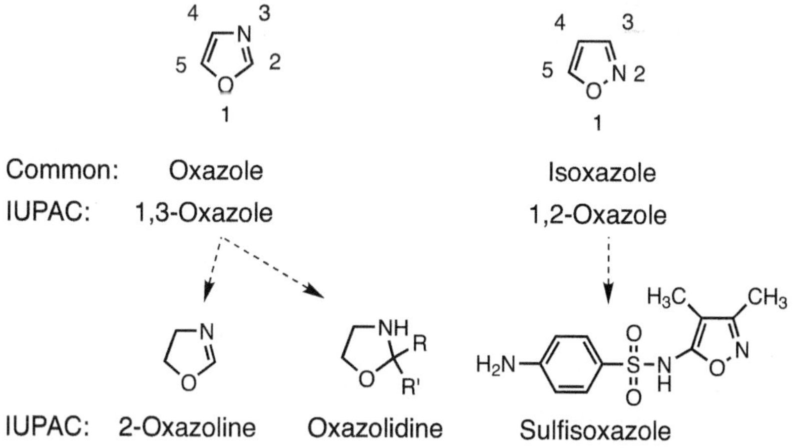

Common: Oxazole   Isoxazole

IUPAC: 1,3-Oxazole   1,2-Oxazole

IUPAC: 2-Oxazoline   Oxazolidine   Sulfisoxazole

FIGURE 15-15. Oxazole and isoxazole heterocycles and derivatives of these heterocycles.

acetal. An explanation of this terminology would appear valuable. As previously discussed (see Chapter 9), an aldehyde or ketone can react with two alcohols under acidic conditions to form an acetal or ketal, respectively (Fig. 9-4). In a similar manner an amine and an alcohol, especially if constituents of the same molecule such as in 1,3-ethanolamine, can react with an aldehyde or ketone under acidic conditions to form a mixed acetal, 2-substituted oxazolidine, or a mixed ketal, 2,2-disubstituted oxazolidine (Fig. 15-16). The "mixed" designation is used to indicate that unlike a typical acetal or ketal that is composed of two oxygen atoms replacing the aldehyde or ketone oxygen, one or more heteroatoms have replaced an oxygen in the acetal or ketal. Sulfur is another heteroatom that can replace oxygen in an acetal or ketal to again give a mixed acetal or mixed ketal. Additionally, both oxygens can be replaced with heteroatoms (N or S) to give "mixed" acetal or ketals (see imidazolidine). Consistent with the chemistry of acetals and ketals is the fact that mixed acetals and mixed ketals are unstable in aqueous acid as shown in Figure 15-18.

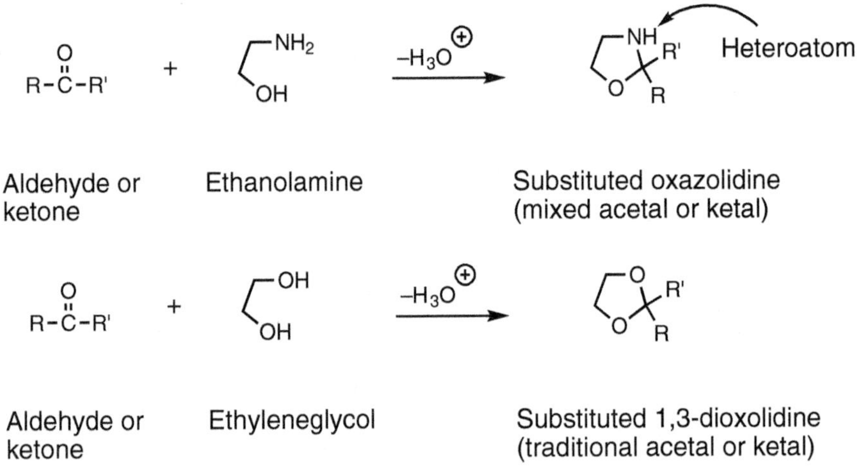

FIGURE 15-16. Acid catalyzed synthesis of a subsituted oxazolidine, mixed acetals, and ketals.

■ **PHYSICAL-CHEMICAL PROPERTIES.** Both oxazole and isoxazole are aromatic compounds. The aromatic π cloud is made up of two electrons from each double bond, plus a pair of electrons contributed by the oxygen atom. Since nitrogen is left with its unshared pair of electrons, both of these compounds are basic, although they should be recognized as weak bases ($pK_a < 6.0$ of the protonated nitrogen) (Fig. 15-17). Both compounds can be converted to salts with a strong acid such as hydrochloric acid. As their hydrochloric salts, oxazoles and isoxazoles would be predicted to be water-soluble.

2-Oxazoline and oxazolidine are also basic compounds but prove unstable in aqueous acid media. An example of such instability is shown in Figure 15-18.

■ **METABOLISM.** The only characteristic metabolism of significance is aromatic hydroxylation. In the case of oxazole, the product formed exists in the "keto" form shown in Figure 15-19.

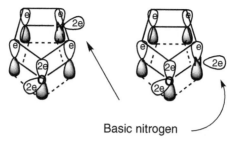

Basic nitrogen

FIGURE 15-17. π Electron structure of oxazole and isoxazole.

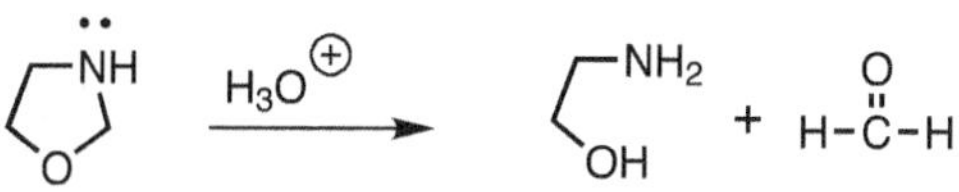

FIGURE 15-18. Acid catalyzed hydrolysis of oxazolidine.

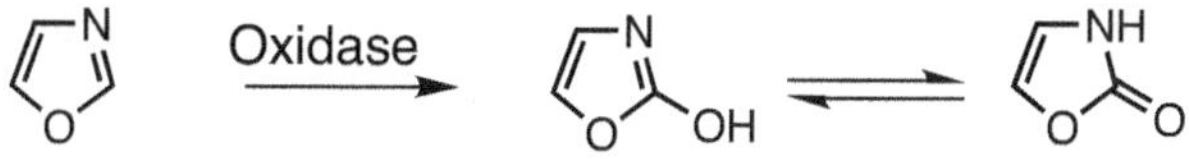

FIGURE 15-19. Metabolic hydroxylation of oxazole.

Nitrogen and Nitrogen

■ **NOMENCLATURE.** Two important dinitrogen heterocycles are found in medicinal agents; these are imidazole and pyrazole (Fig. 15-20). As with several previous examples, the student should be familiar with the common name, since it is used in most cases. The important partially reduced and saturated analogs of imidazole are 2-imidazoline and imidazolidine, respectively. These compounds are numbered similarly to that shown for imidazole.

There are a variety of imidazole-containing drugs but far fewer pyrazole-containing agents.

■ **PHYSICAL-CHEMICAL PROPERTIES.** Pyrazole and imidazole are both aromatic compounds that have one basic nitrogen and a neutral nitrogen. The aromatic nature arises from the four π electrons and the unshared pair of electrons on the -NH- nitrogen. Some care should be taken in specifying which nitrogen is basic since, in unsymmetrical derivatives, resonance prevents one from isolating a specific compound, as shown in Figure 15-21. All that can be said is that one nitrogen is basic.

In 2-imidazoline, both nitrogens are basic. The 2° amine is more basic than the sp^2 nitrogen, but again it may not be possible to specify which is sp^3 and which is sp^2. Imidazolidine, on the other hand, is made up of two 2° amines and is quite basic. Imidazolidine, like oxazolidine, is unstable in aqueous acid and is hydrolyzed to ethylenediamine and formaldehyde (Fig. 15-22). This again is related to the fact

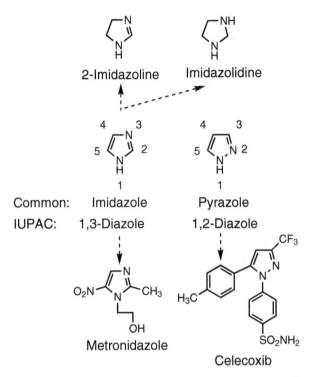

FIGURE 15-20. Imidazole and pyrazole heterocycles, reduction products of imidazole, and derivatives of imidazole and pyrazole.

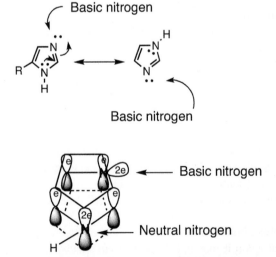

FIGURE 15-21. The imidazole heterocycle has one basic nitrogen, which, because of resonance, may be either nitrogen.

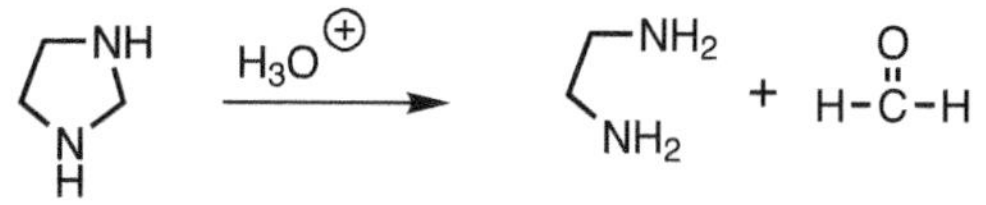

FIGURE 15-22. Acid catalyzed hydrolysis of imidazolidine.

that imidazolidine is an acetal derivative, in which both oxygens of a typical acetal are replaced with nitrogens.

▪ **METABOLISM.** The predicted metabolism is uneventful. While the aromatic compounds may be prone to hydroxylation, the reduced heterocycles would be expected to act like secondary amines in vivo and undergo conjugation reactions.

Nitrogen and Sulfur

▪ **NOMENCLATURE.** The only heterocycle to be considered that contains a nitrogen and sulfur in a five-membered ring is the chemical 1,3-thiazole (Fig. 15-23). The nomenclature used is that derived from Tables 15-1 and 15-2. The thiazole nucleus is a very common moiety found in many drug molecules.

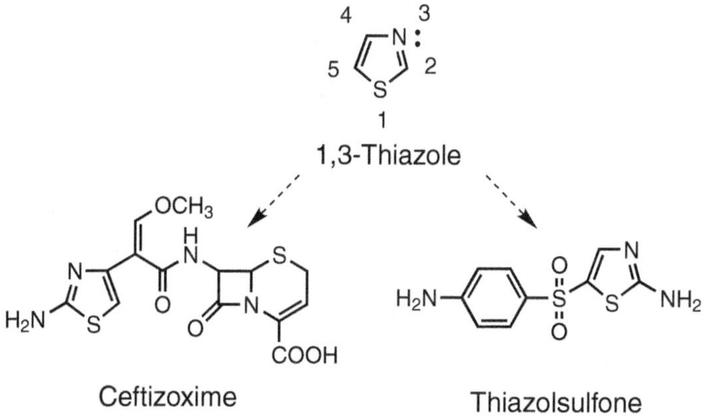

FIGURE 15-23. Structure of 1,3-thiazole and examples of drugs containing this nucleus.

▪ **PHYSICAL-CHEMICAL PROPERTIES.** The properties of thiazole are similar to those of oxazole. This compound is aromatic, and the nitrogen in this compound with its unshared pair of electrons is weakly basic (pK_a 2.44).

▪ **METABOLISM.** The metabolic properties are analogous to those of the other aromatic heterocycles and consist of aromatic hydroxylation at any of the carbon hydrogen locations.

Complex Five-Membered Heterocycles

▪ **NOMENCLATURE.** A series of miscellaneous heterocycles important to medicinal chemistry are shown in this section, along with a few examples of drugs containing these heterocycles. The 1,3,4-thiadiazole and 1,2,5-thiadiazole have nomenclature that is self-explanatory and follows the priority rules previously mentioned and the abbreviations for the heteroatoms (a sulfur, two nitrogens in a five-membered ring) (Fig. 15-24).

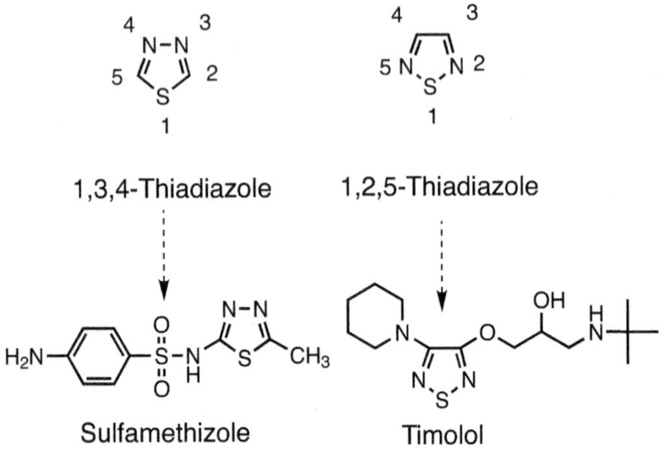

FIGURE 15-24. Structure of thiadiazoles and examples of drugs containing this nucleus.

Several triazoles exist, in which the "tri" indicates three, "az" signifies nitrogen, and "ole" indicates a five-membered ring (Fig. 15-25). If the three nitrogens are symmetrically arranged (at the 1, 3, and 4 positions), the compound can be identified as s-Triazole ("s" for symmetrical), while if not symmetrically arranged the compound is named 1H-1,2,4-triazole. One additional poly nitrogen-containing heterocycle is tetrazole.

The oxazolidinone and oxazolidinedione nomenclature should be understandable based on the oxazolidine nomenclature explained earlier, with the "one" signifying a carbonyl and "dione" representing two carbonyls at the 2 and 4 positions (Fig. 15-26).

One additional important heterocycle is the hydantoin nucleus. Here the common nomenclature replaces the official nomenclature of imidazolidinedione. A number of very important classes of drugs possess these heterocyclic nuclei.

■ **PHYSICAL-CHEMICAL PROPERTIES.** The thiadiazoles, triazoles, and tetrazoles are typical aromatic nuclei that have two (thiadiazole, triazole) or three (tetrazole) basic nitrogens in the ring. If one accounts for the electrons required for aromaticity, it should be obvious which nitrogens retain the electrons necessary for basicity, although the triazoles are weak bases ($pK_a \sim 1-2$). Little additional information is necessary, since none of these compounds has any unique physical-chemical properties that one needs to be concerned with.

The oxazolidin-2-ones are cyclic analogs of a class of compounds discussed previously, namely the carbamates. Like their straight-chain relatives, the oxazolidin-2-ones are readily hydrolyzed by acid or basic media (Fig. 15-27).

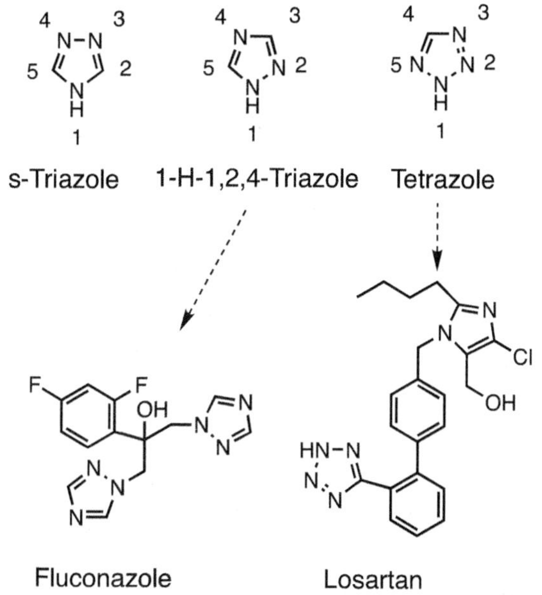

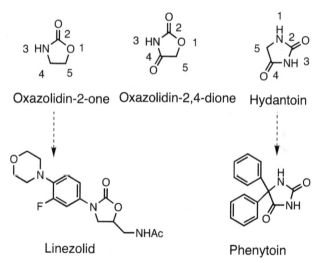

s-Triazole   1-H-1,2,4-Triazole   Tetrazole

Fluconazole   Losartan

FIGURE 15-25. Structure of triazoles and tetrazole, and examples of drugs containing these nuclei.

Oxazolidin-2-one   Oxazolidin-2,4-dione   Hydantoin

Linezolid   Phenytoin

FIGURE 15-26. Structure of oxazolidinones, hydantoin and examples of drugs containing these nuclei.

The oxazolidin-2,4-diones do have a chemical property unique to the "imide" portion of the structure (Fig. 15-28). Although an amide is neutral, the addition of a second carbonyl covalently bonded to the nitrogen produces the imide functional group, which has acidic properties provided the nitrogen has an attached hydrogen.

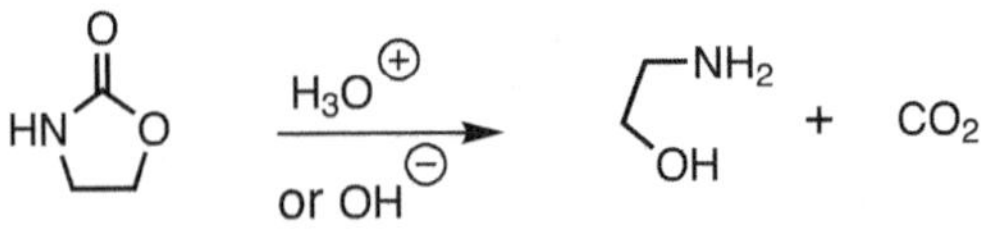

FIGURE 15-27. Acid- or base-catalyzed hydrolysis of oxazolidin-2-one.

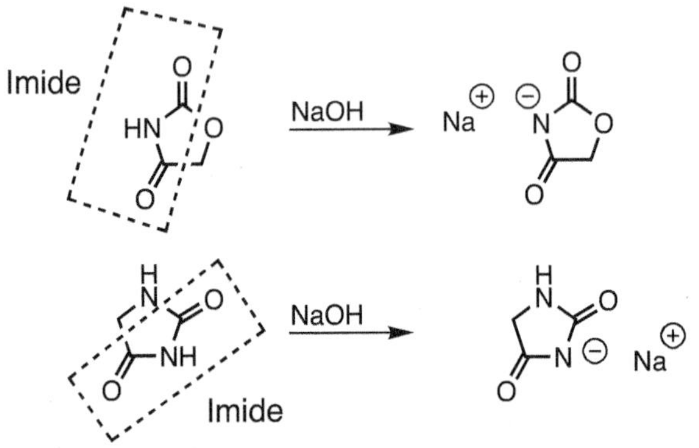

FIGURE 15-28. Salt formation at the imide nitrogen of oxazolidin-2,4-dione and hydantoin.

Two electron-withdrawing groups on either side of the -NH- group withdraw the unshared pair of electrons on the nitrogen as well as the electron pair remaining after dissociation of the hydrogen. This allows the hydrogen to be abstracted by a strong base, forming an alkaline salt that is quite water-soluble.

The final heterocycle, the hydantoin, is a cyclic urea, but in addition it contains an imide functional group. The presence of the hydrogen on the imide nitrogen again results in a compound with acidic properties.

SIX-MEMBERED RING HETEROCYCLES

Nitrogen

■ **NOMENCLATURE.** The important six-membered ring nitrogen-containing heterocycles are pyridine, the aromatic compound, and piperidine, the saturated compound (Fig. 15-29). While both common and IUPAC nomenclature is shown, in most cases the common name is used exclusively. These two heterocycles are commonly found in a variety of medicinal agents.

■ **PHYSICAL-CHEMICAL PROPERTIES.** Pyridine, unlike its carbon analog benzene, is quite water-soluble. The explanation for this fact lies in the availability of an unshared pair of electrons found on the nitrogen. This polar compound can hydrogen bond to water through this pair of electrons. The availability of the electrons accounts for the other property of pyridine that makes it different from pyrrole,

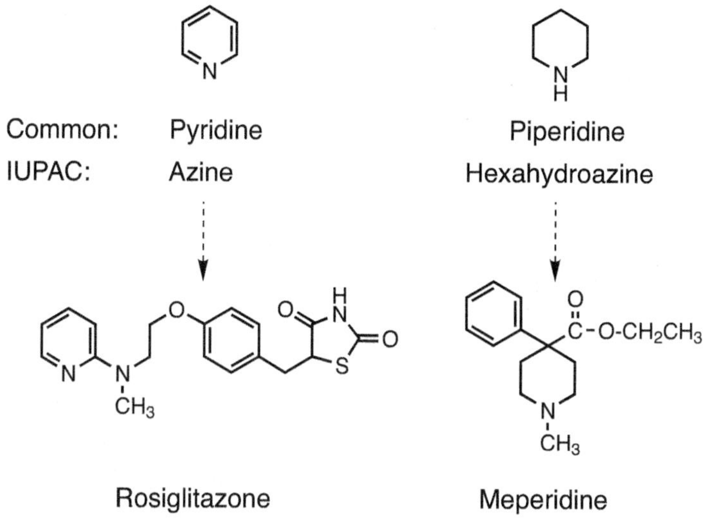

FIGURE 15-29. Structure of pyridine, piperidine, and examples of drugs containing these nuclei.

namely the basicity of pyridine. Pyridinium ion has a pK_a of 5.36, which can be compared with the nearly neutral pyrrole's pK_a of 0.398, yet pyridine is much less basic than alkylamines, which have pK_a's of approximately 10 for the alkylammonium ions. Pyridine and substituted pyridines have approximately the same basicity as the aromatic ammonium ions such as aniline (pK_a of 4.6). Thus, it would be difficult to predict a difference in basicity between the two nitrogens in the following compound:

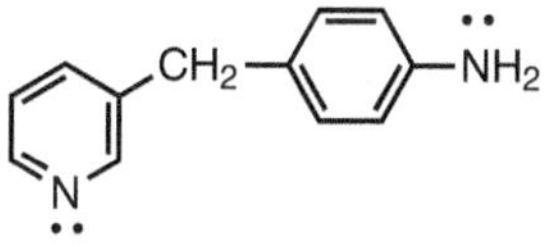

On the other hand, piperidine is nothing more than a cyclic alkyl amine. It is quite basic, with a $pK_a \approx 11.3$ for the piperidinium ion. Other than the reactivity of pyridine and piperidine toward strong acids, one should consider both of these compounds as relatively stable.

■ METABOLISM. Pyridine, since it is an aromatic compound, acts like the typical aromatic rings and undergoes hydroxylation. Piperidine acts like a typical secondary amine and would be predicted to undergo conjugation with glucuronic acid or sulfuric acid.

Dealkylation resulting in ring cleavage would not be expected to occur with piperidine, since dealkylation occurs primarily with amines that are substituted with smaller alkyl groups such as methyl or ethyl groups.

SIX-MEMBERED RING HETEROCYCLES WITH TWO HETEROATOMS

Nitrogen and Nitrogen

■ **NOMENCLATURE.** Several important heterocycles are formed from two nitrogens in a six-membered ring, and these are shown here with their respective nomenclature (Fig. 15-30). Once again, the official nomenclature is usually neglected in favor of common nomenclature.

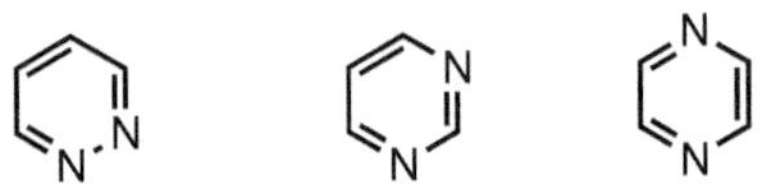

Common:	Pyridazine	Pyrimidine	Pyrazine
IUPAC:	1,2-Diazine	1,3-Diazine	1,4-Diazine
pHa (protonated heterocycle)	2.24	1.23	0.65

FIGURE 15-30. Structures of the isomer diazines.

■ **PHYSICAL-CHEMICAL PROPERTIES.** All three of the compounds shown in Figure 15-30 have properties similar to each other and similar to the properties of pyridine. The compounds are basic with varying pK_as. Since these compounds are aromatic, they are also expected to be relatively nonreactive. Finally, parallel to the solubility properties of pyridine, these compounds are also water-soluble.

Pyrimidines—I

■ **NOMENCLATURE.** Three pyrimidine derivatives that are important to the structure of DNA and RNA, as well as to the structure of medicinally active agents, are shown in Figure 15-31. While official nomenclature can be derived for these compounds, it is replaced with the common names presented. Thymine may also be referred to as 5-methyluracil. It is important to recognize the numbering system of these heterocycles. A clockwise direction is chosen such that the heteroatoms appear at the 1 and 3 positions and the carbonyls or carbonyl and amine are at the 2 and 4 positions, respectively. If the numbering were counterclockwise, the substituents on the ring would be at the 2 and 6 positions. The pyrimidine nucleus is especially important in anticancer and antiviral drugs.

■ **PHYSICAL-CHEMICAL PROPERTIES.** The substituted pyrimidines are complex molecules because of the nature of the substituents. Uracil and thymine may be considered to contain the neutral urea unit or the acidic imide moiety, as shown in Figure 15-32, but they can also be considered to exist in either the "keto" form or "enol" form, as shown in Figure 15-33. The "enol" form would be expected to have the acidic properties of a diphenolic compound and the basic properties of a

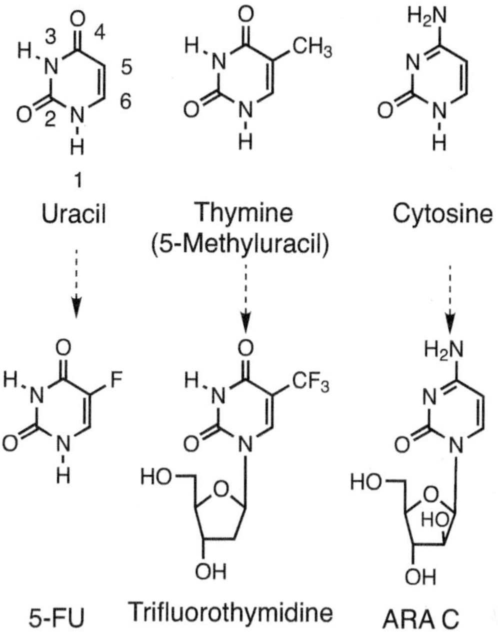

FIGURE 15-31. Structures of functionalized pyrimidines and examples of drugs containing these nuclei.

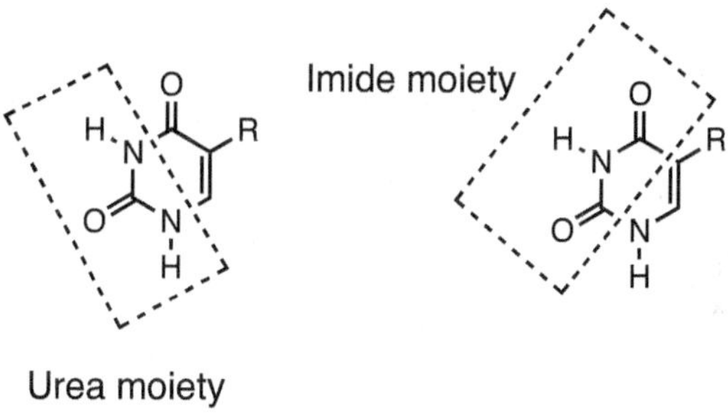

FIGURE 15-32. Structural units of the uracil nucleus.

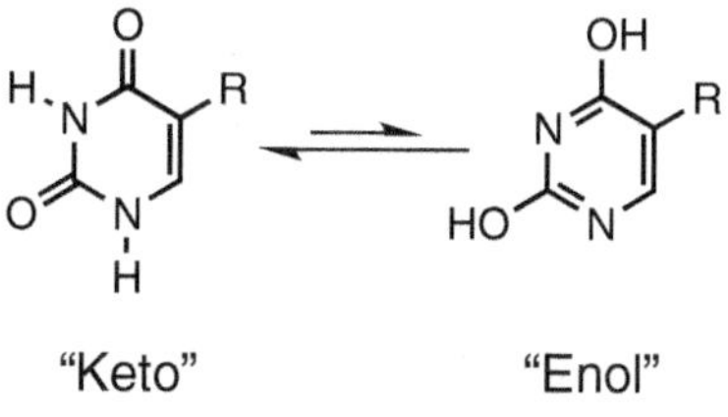

FIGURE 15-33. "Keto"–"enol" equilibrium of the uracil ring.

pyrimidine. Since the compounds prefer the "keto" form, they are usually thought of as weak acids, but the weak acid-weak base properties of the "enol" form may account for the reduced solubility in water of uracil and thymine. Cytosine, with the 4-amino substituent and without an imide moiety, might be expected to be a weak base.

None of the substituted pyrimidines has any noteworthy instabilities.

■ **METABOLISM.** The metabolism of these unique pyrimidines is important from the standpoint of both biochemical utilization of these compounds and drug metabolism of pyrimidine derivatives. Figure 15-34 outlines a pathway that converts uracil to a useful compound, uridylic acid, needed for the synthesis of RNA.

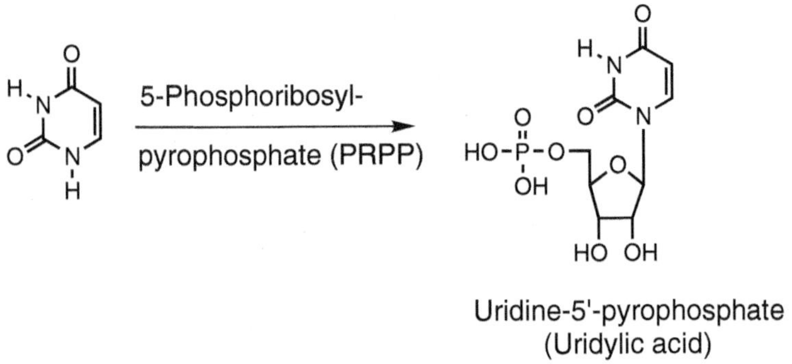

Uridine-5'-pyrophosphate
(Uridylic acid)

FIGURE 15-34. Metabolism of uracil.

In a similar manner to that shown for uracil, cytosine is conjugated with PRPP to yield cytidine-5'-monophosphate (CMP) or cytidylic acid. Thymine is metabolized by conjugation, via a salvage pathway, with PRPP to the thymine ribosyl-5'-phosphate. This form of thymidylic acid can be utilized in specific RNA molecules. The biochemically important thymine deoxyribosyl-5'-phosphate is important in the biosynthesis of DNA but is derived from uridylic acid, which is first converted to deoxyuridylic acid and then into the deoxythymidylic acid (Fig. 15-35).

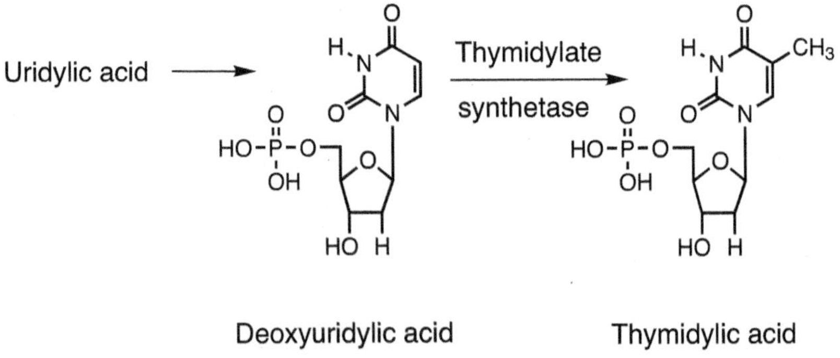

Deoxyuridylic acid   Thymidylic acid

FIGURE 15-35. Biosynthesis of thymidylic acid.

An example of a pyrimidine-substituted drug and its metabolic pattern is shown in Figure 15-36. 5-Fluorouracil can be conjugated with either ribose or deoxyribose, and the sugar is then phosphorylated to either 5-fluorouridine monophosphate (5-FUMP) or 5-fluorouridine-2'-deoxyribosyl phosphate (5-FUDR). In this particular example, the 5-FUMP is responsible for the side effects of the drug, while 5-FUDR is responsible for the chemotherapeutic action of 5-FU. 5-FU is an example of an administered drug that must be "activated"; that is, it must be converted to an active drug to produce its intended pharmacologic action. Drugs such as 5-FU are referred to as "pro-drugs" since they come before the actual "active" drug (5-FUDR).

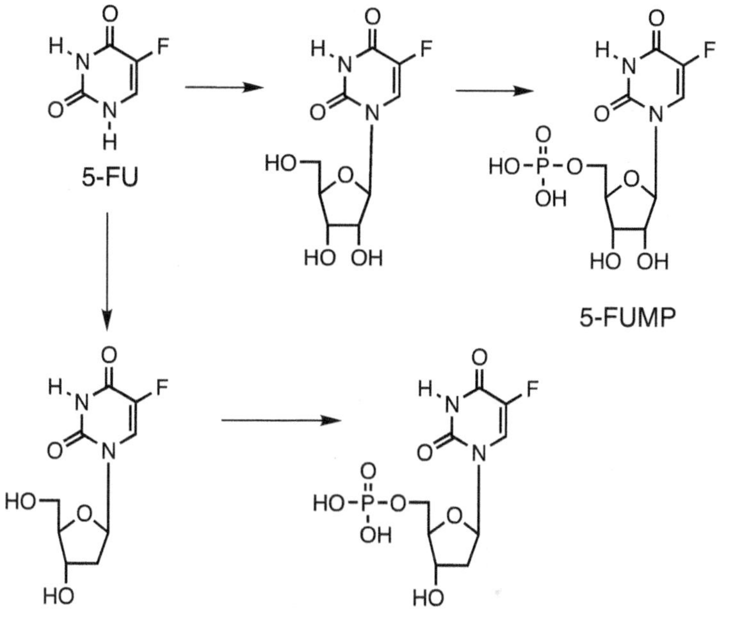

FIGURE 15-36. Metabolism of 5-fluorouracil.

Pyrimidines—II

■ **NOMENCLATURE.** Two additional special pyrimidines are barbituric acid and the substituted barbiturates (Fig. 15-37). The substituted barbiturates represent a special class of compounds that have been used for their sedative-hypnotic action since the early 1900s. The numbering system starts with either nitrogen and proceeds such that the substituents (R) appear at the 5 position.

■ **PHYSICAL-CHEMICAL PROPERTIES.** Barbituric acid can exist in any of the four forms shown in Figure 15-38. Roentgenographic studies have shown that as a solid, the compound exists in the trioxo form, while in solution evidence rules against the trihydroxy form but supports the presence of the other enolic forms.

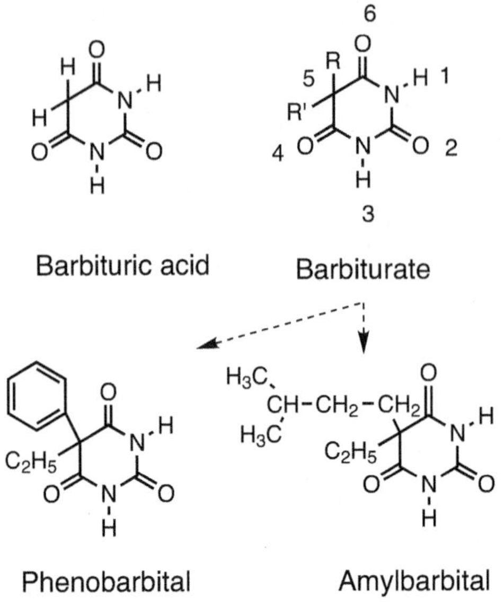

Barbituric acid   Barbiturate

Phenobarbital   Amylbarbital

FIGURE 15-37. Structure of barbituric acid and examples of drugs containing the barbiturate nucleus.

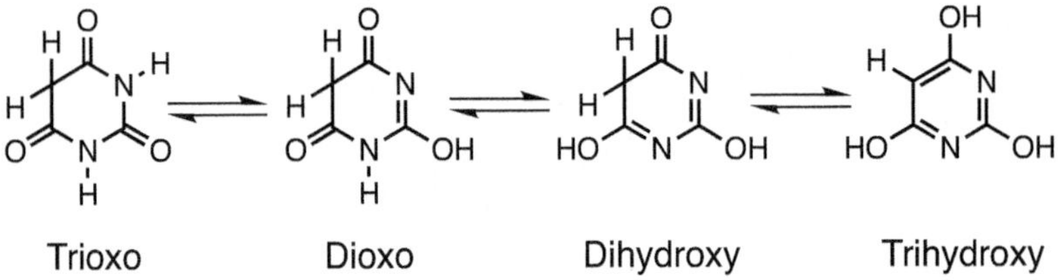

Trioxo   Dioxo   Dihydroxy   Trihydroxy

FIGURE 15-38. "Keto"–"enol" equilibrium of barbituric acid.

Barbituric acid is a fairly strong acid with a pK_a of 4.12, but upon substitution at the 5 position, the pK_a rises dramatically. The 5,5-disubstituted barbiturates have pK_a values of 7.1 to 8.1. Such compounds exist predominantly in the trioxo tautomeric form (Fig. 15-39). The 5,5-disubstituted barbiturates react with sodium hydroxide to form a salt that is quite water-soluble (Fig. 15-40). Such salts, when

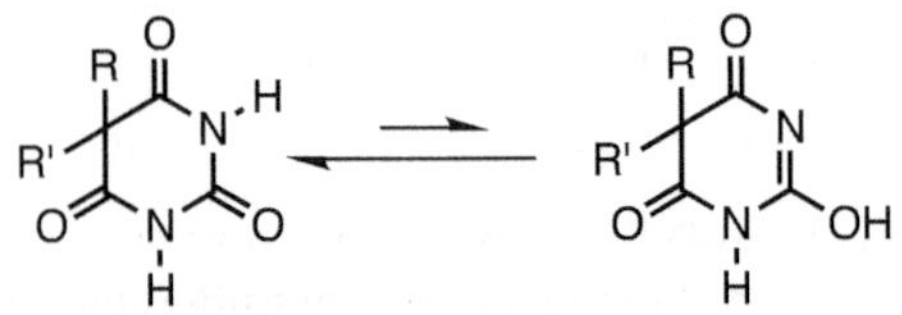

FIGURE 15-39. "Keto"–"enol" equilibrium of 5,5-disubstituted barbituric acids.

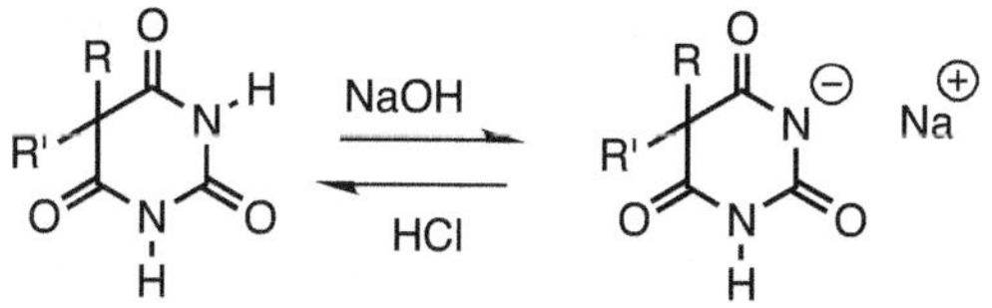

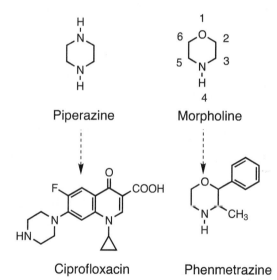

FIGURE 15-40. Salt formation of 5,5-disubstituted barbituric acids.

added to water, result in an aqueous medium that becomes quite alkaline owing to the fact that such a salt is made up of a weak acid and a strong base. If the pH of the medium is titrated to a neutral or acidic pH, the reaction will be reversed, resulting in precipitation of barbituric acid.

SATURATED SIX-MEMBERED RING HETEROCYCLES

■ **NOMENCLATURE.** Two important saturated heterocycles that appear in drug molecules are piperazine and morpholine (Fig. 15-41). The common names are used in nearly all cases when referring to these nuclei.

Piperazine   Morpholine

Ciprofloxacin   Phenmetrazine

FIGURE 15-41. Structure of piperazine, morpholine, and examples of drugs containing these nuclei.

■ **PHYSICAL-CHEMICAL PROPERTIES.** Since these compounds are cyclic forms of a diamine, piperazine, and a secondary amine plus an ether, morpholine, the properties are the same as those reviewed in the chapters on these respective functional groups and need not be discussed at this point.

SEVEN- AND EIGHT-MEMBERED RING HETEROCYCLES

Nitrogen

■ **NOMENCLATURE.** Two heterocycles that complete our review of monocyclic heterocycles are hexahydroazepine and octahydroazocine (Fig. 15-42). The fully reduced azepine and azocine appear in a number of medicinal agents, and in addition the azepine is part of a tricyclic ring system that will be discussed later in the chapter.

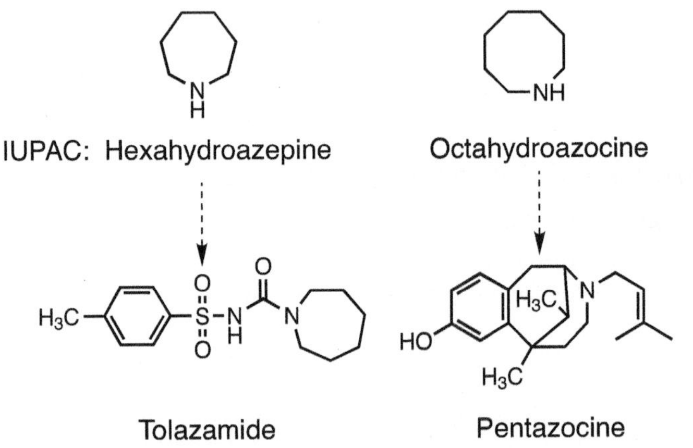

IUPAC: Hexahydroazepine   Octahydroazocine

Tolazamide   Pentazocine

FIGURE 15-42. Structure of hexahydroazepine, octahydroazocine, and an example of a drug containing the hydroazocine nucleus.

■ **PHYSICAL-CHEMICAL PROPERTIES.** Both hexahydroazepine and octahydroazocine are cyclic secondary amines that are basic compounds and act like ordinary alkylamines.

BICYCLIC HETEROCYCLES: FIVE-MEMBERED RING PLUS SIX-MEMBERED RING

One Nitrogen

■ **NOMENCLATURE.** An important bicyclic ring system containing a single nitrogen is indole. This nucleus is present in the amino acid tryptophan and is found in many alkaloids. Less important from a medicinal standpoint is the isomer of indole, isoindole (Fig. 15-43).

■ **PHYSICAL-CHEMICAL PROPERTIES.** Indole is an aromatic compound with delocalization of the electrons across both rings (Fig. 15-44). Thus, like pyrrole, the benzopyrroles require the unshared pair of electrons on nitrogen to participate in the delocalized cloud of electrons. The result of this delocalization is that indole is a weak base and for our purposes will be considered neutral.

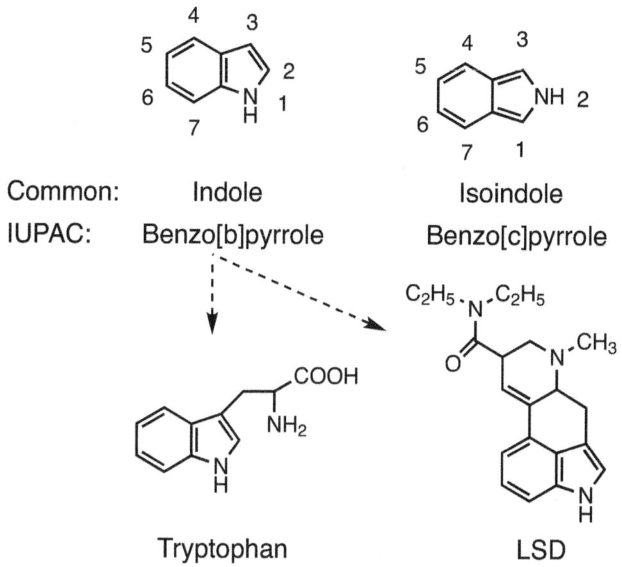

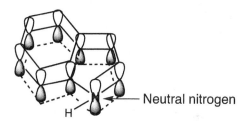

Common: Indole   Isoindole

IUPAC: Benzo[b]pyrrole   Benzo[c]pyrrole

Tryptophan   LSD

FIGURE 15-43. Structure of indole, isoindole, and examples of compounds containing these nuclei.

Neutral nitrogen

FIGURE 15-44. π Electron structure of indole.

Indole and drugs containing the indole nucleus are easily oxidized when allowed to stand in contact with air. An indication of this reaction is the darkening of the color of the compound. It is best if indole-containing drugs are protected from atmospheric oxygen by storing under nitrogen.

▪ **METABOLISM.** Since indole is an aromatic nucleus, it is expected that aromatic hydroxylation would occur. Most indole-containing drugs are substituted at the 3 position, and the hydroxylation occurs at the 4–7 position of the molecule.

Two Heteroatoms

▪ **NOMENCLATURE.** Three bicyclic heterocycles that contain two heteroatoms are shown in Figure 15-45. The common nomenclature is based upon the name of the five-membered ring, and since it is fused to a benzene ring, they are

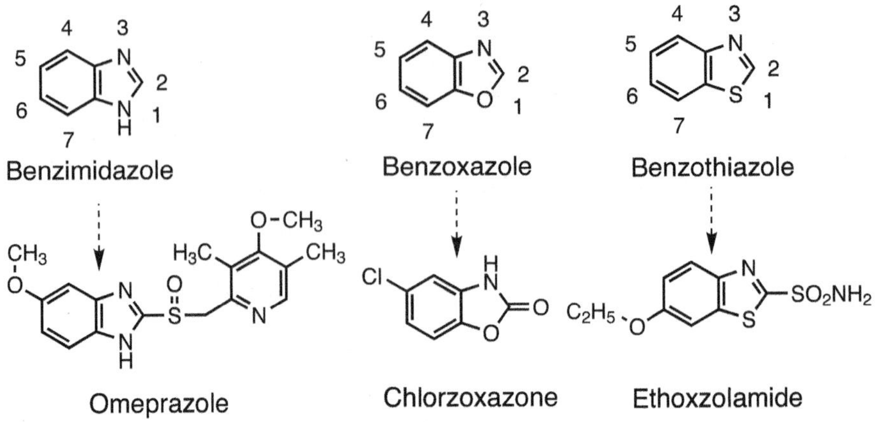

FIGURE 15-45. Structures of benzimidazole, benzoxazole, benzothiazole, and examples of drugs containing these nuclei.

referred to as benz(o) ("o" is dropped when followed by a vowel) and then the name of the five-membered ring heterocycle. The numbering proceeds as shown. The bridgehead positions (e.g., the positions where the two rings join) are not numbered because the carbons at the bridgehead are already fully substituted. In cases in which the benzene ring is reduced, the bridgehead position can be numbered at the 3a and 7a positions since they follow the 3 and 7 positions, respectively.

■ **PHYSICAL-CHEMICAL PROPERTIES.** The properties of the benzimidazole, benzoxazole, and benzothiazole do not differ significantly from the properties of imidazole, oxazole, or thiazole. All three compounds are aromatic, and all three have a weakly basic nitrogen in the molecule. The only property that does change is the fact that the molecules are less water-soluble, since each has four additional carbon atoms present.

■ **METABOLISM.** The predicted metabolism of these heterocycles is aromatic hydroxylation. The hydroxylation can occur at any of the positions occupied by hydrogen (2, 4, 5, 6, or 7 positions).

Four Heteroatoms

■ **NOMENCLATURE.** An important bicyclic heterocycle is the purine nucleus (Fig. 15-46). The purine can be thought of as a pyrimidine fused to an imidazole. The numbering follows this type of analogy. The six-membered ring is numbered first, starting with one nitrogen atom and proceeding counterclockwise completely around the ring, including the bridgehead positions. This is then followed by numbering the five-membered ring.

Three common substituted purines should be familiar to the reader and are also shown in Figure 15-46. They include the 6-aminopurine (adenine), 2-amino-6-hydroxypurine (guanine) (which actually exists not in the "enol" but rather in the

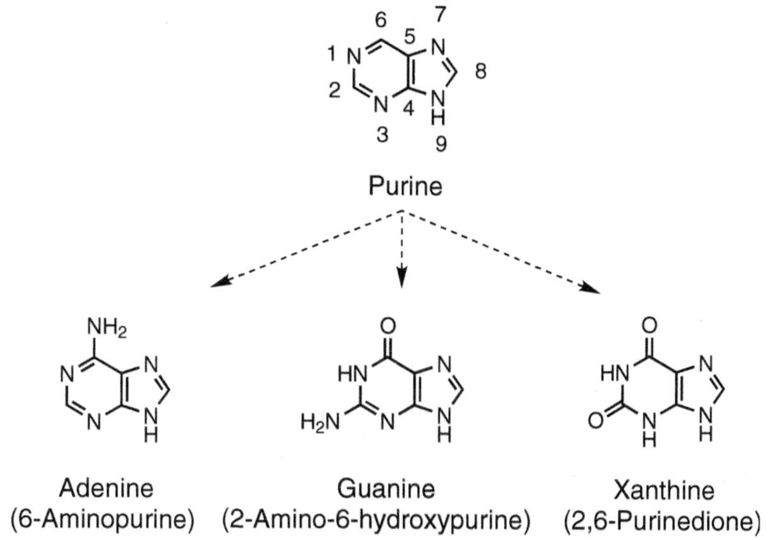

Purine

Adenine   Guanine   Xanthine
(6-Aminopurine)   (2-Amino-6-hydroxypurine)   (2,6-Purinedione)

FIGURE 15-46. Structures of purine and the biologically significant substituted purines.

"keto" form), and 2,6-purinedione (xanthine). All three of these compounds are common metabolites found in the human body and are important nuclei in a number of drug molecules.

■ **PHYSICAL-CHEMICAL PROPERTIES.** Purine is an aromatic compound containing three basic nitrogens. Because of the ability of this compound to hydrogen bond to water through the unshared pair of electrons on the nitrogens, the compound is highly soluble in water. With functionalization of the purine ring, as in the case of adenine, guanine, and xanthine, the water solubility decreases. This is probably due to intramolecular interactions, which is discussed in Chapter 18. Let it suffice to say that intramolecular interactions such as those shown in Figure 15-47 decrease the attractions that can occur with water. Finally, xanthine has both basic

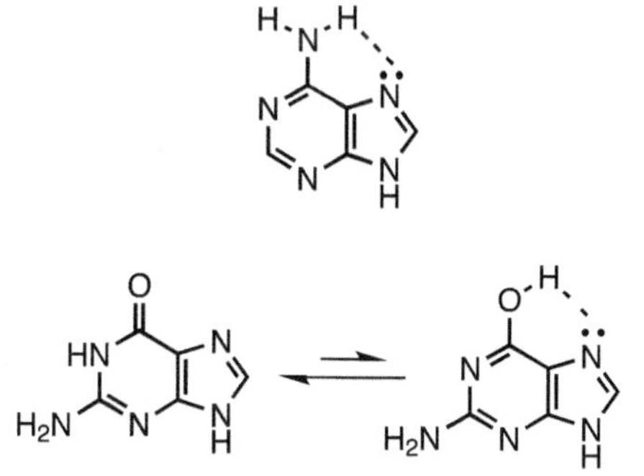

FIGURE 15-47. Intramolecular bonding present in adenine and guanine.

properties due to one of the nitrogens in the imidazole ring and acidic properties due to the imide NH in the pyrimidine ring.

■ **METABOLISM.** The metabolism of the substituted purine is quite systematic and is shown for adenine in Figure 15-48. The adenine is conjugated with 5-phosphoribosylpyrophosphate (PRPP) to give adenylic acid (adenosine-5'-phosphate). Adenylic acid in turn may be reduced to deoxyadenylic acid. A similar pattern of metabolism can lead to guanosine and xanthosine, which in turn can lead to guanylic acid and xanthylic acid.

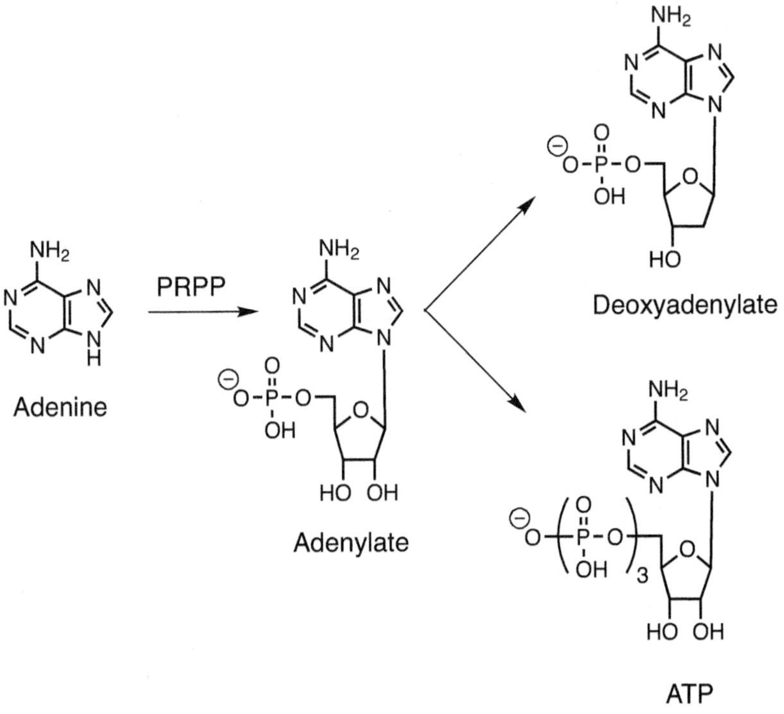

FIGURE 15-48. Metabolism of adenine.

A second type of metabolism common to purines is aromatic hydroxylation. An enzyme known as xanthine oxidase catalyzes this reaction. When xanthine is oxidized by xanthine oxidase, the resulting product is uric acid (Fig. 15-49).

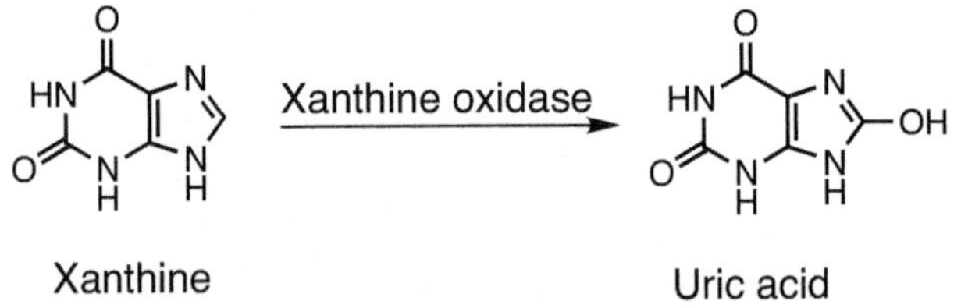

Xanthine · Xanthine oxidase · Uric acid

FIGURE 15-49. Metabolism of xanthine.

BICYCLIC HETEROCYCLES: SIX-MEMBERED RING PLUS SIX-MEMBERED RING

One Nitrogen

■ **NOMENCLATURE.** Two important bicyclic heterocycles containing a nitrogen in two fused six-membered rings are quinoline and isoquinoline (Fig. 15-50). These nuclei are common to synthetic and naturally occurring drugs. The rings are numbered as shown. The bridgehead positions are not numbered.

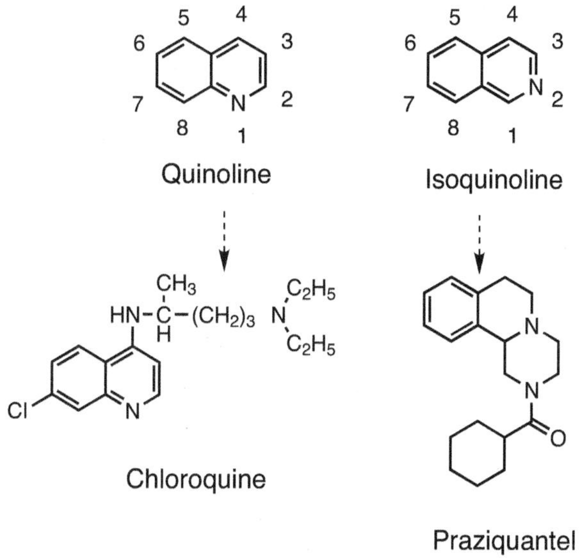

FIGURE 15-50. Structures of quinoline, isoquinoline, and examples of drugs containing these nuclei.

■ **PHYSICAL-CHEMICAL PROPERTIES.** Both quinoline and isoquinoline are weak bases similar to pyridine. These weak bases react with a strong acid such as sulfuric acid or hydrochloric acid to form water-soluble salts ($pK_a \sim 5.0$). Both compounds are aromatic and therefore have few additional properties that need concern us.

■ **METABOLISM.** The common metabolism seen in quinolines and isoquinolines is aromatic hydroxylation at one of the positions occupied by hydrogen.

One Oxygen

■ **NOMENCLATURE.** Another important bicyclic heterocycle found in nature and several synthetic drugs is the coumarin molecule (Fig. 15-51). Although the compound possesses a more complicated official name, the common name is usually used.

■ **PHYSICAL-CHEMICAL PROPERTIES.** The coumarin molecule contains an intramolecular ester known as a lactone. Lactones experience the same types of

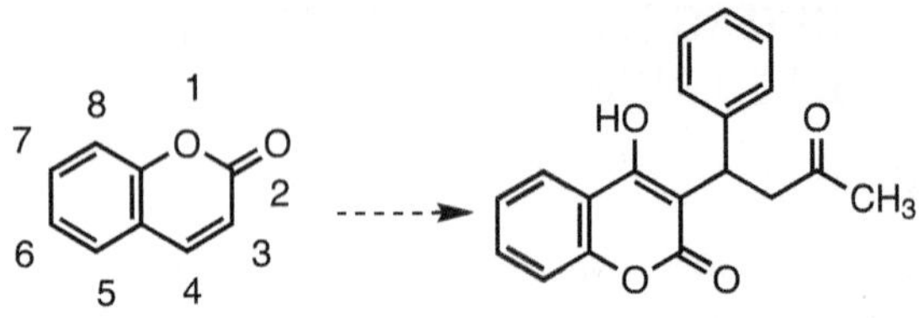

Common: Coumarin   Warfarin

IUPAC: 2H-Benzopyran-2-one

FIGURE 15-51. Structure of coumarin and an example of a drug containing the coumarin nucleus.

instabilities as esters. Lactones are prone to hydrolysis catalyzed by either acid or base to give a carboxylic acid and phenol (Fig. 15-52) (see Chapter 12 and Fig. 12-2).

■ **METABOLISM.** Esterase-catalyzed hydrolysis of coumarins would be expected to occur in the body, the product being the more soluble carboxylic acid shown in Figure 15-52.

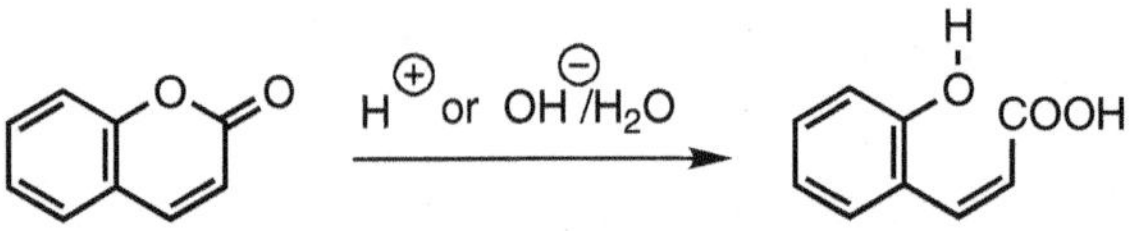

FIGURE 15-52. Acid- or base-catalyzed hydrolysis of coumarin.

Two or More Nitrogens

■ **NOMENCLATURE.** Two additional bicyclic heterocycles that serve as nuclei for several synthetic drugs and natural products are quinazoline and pteridine (Fig. 15-53).

■ **PHYSICAL-CHEMICAL PROPERTIES.** The properties of quinazoline and pteridine are similar to the monocyclic six-membered heterocycles. Both compounds are aromatic and possess basic nitrogens. Like pyridine or pyrimidine, the nitrogens are weak bases and therefore form salts in the presence of a strong acid.

■ **METABOLISM.** The metabolism expected for both quinazoline and pteridine is aromatic hydroxylation. This can occur at any of the positions occupied by a hydrogen.

Two Nitrogens Plus Sulfur

■ **NOMENCLATURE.** While there are many additional bicyclic six-plus-six heterocyclics containing a variety of heteroatoms with various arrangements of the

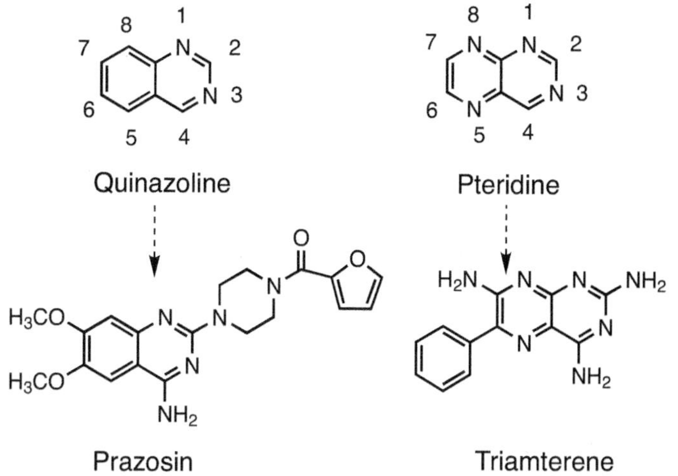

Quinazoline   Pteridine

Prazosin   Triamterene

FIGURE 15-53. Structure of quinazoline, pteridine, and examples of drugs containing these heterocycles.

heteroatoms, one additional nucleus worth mentioning is the benzothiadiazine-1,1-dioxide shown in Figure 15-54. This nucleus is important as it serves as the base for the thiazide diuretics.

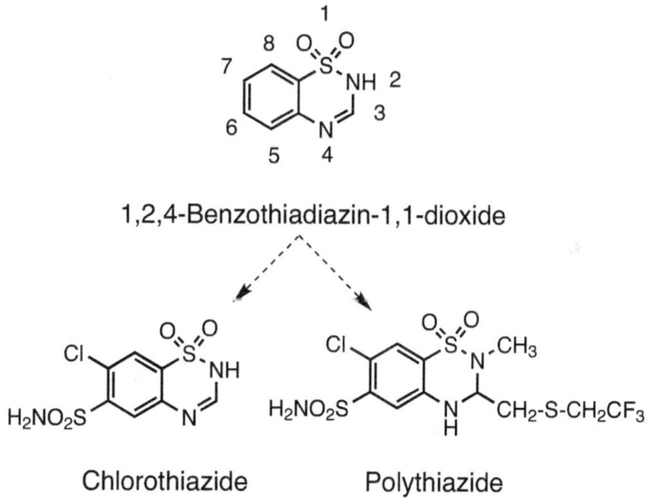

1,2,4-Benzothiadiazin-1,1-dioxide

Chlorothiazide   Polythiazide

FIGURE 15-54. Structure of benzothiadiazinedioxide and examples of drugs containing this heterocycle.

▪ **PHYSICAL-CHEMICAL PROPERTIES.** A recognition of the functionality of this nucleus dictates the properties of the molecule. Present in the benzothiadiazine are a basic nitrogen and a cyclic sulfonamide (Fig. 15-55). The basic nitrogen is a

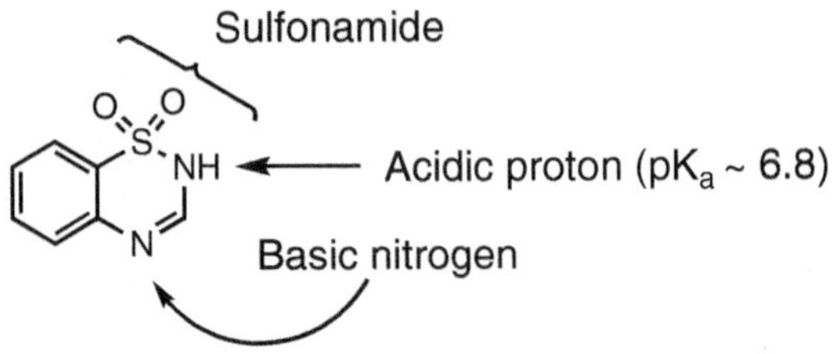

FIGURE 15-55. Functional groups and properties of a thiazide nucleus.

relatively weak base. Depending on whether the sulfonamide nitrogen is substituted or not determines whether this group is acidic or neutral. The unsubstituted sulfonamide nitrogen imparts acidic properties, while substitution at this nitrogen removes the acidic characteristics.

■ **METABOLISM.** No unique metabolic properties are found with this nucleus.

BICYCLIC HETEROCYCLES: SIX-MEMBERED RING PLUS SEVEN-MEMBERED RING

Two Nitrogen Atoms

■ **NOMENCLATURE.** An important six-plus-seven fused bicyclic heterocycle will be encountered in medicinal chemistry. This system is referred to generically as the benzodiazepine class of drugs (Fig. 15-56). The official nomenclature indicates that

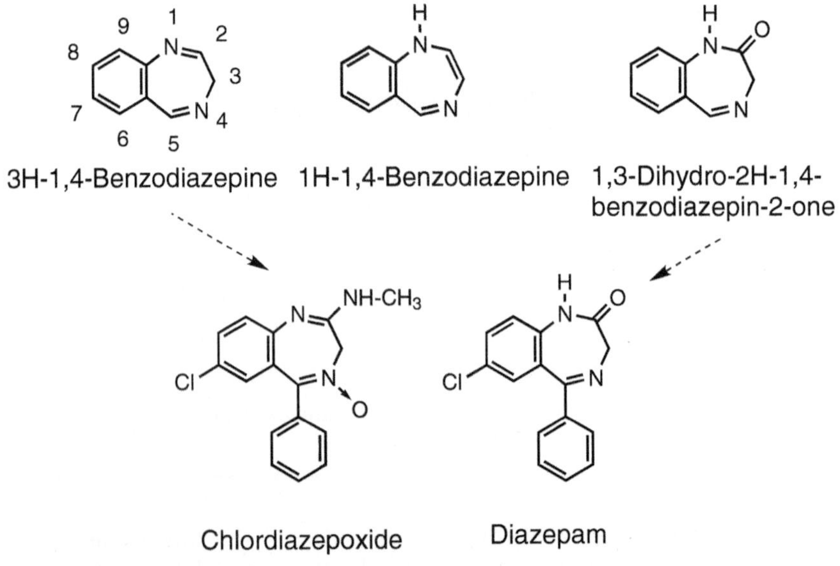

3H-1,4-Benzodiazepine   1H-1,4-Benzodiazepine   1,3-Dihydro-2H-1,4-benzodiazepin-2-one

Chlordiazepoxide   Diazepam

FIGURE 15-56. Structure of 1,4-benzodiazepines and examples of drugs containing this heterocycle.

a benzene ring ("benzo") has been fused to a seven-membered ring ("pine"), which in turn contains two nitrogens ("diaz"). The 1,4- designates the location of the two nitrogen atoms. Since a seven-membered ring can accommodate only three double bonds, the 3H tells indirectly that with a hydrogen at the 3 position, the double bonds are at the site of ring fusion as well as at the 1,2 and 4,5 positions. An alternate arrangement of double bonds is shown for 1H-1,4-benzodiazepine. While 3H-1,4-benzodiazepine is the basic nucleus for the drug chlordiazepoxide, most of the benzodiazepines fall into the class of 1,3-dihydro-2H-1,4-benzodiazepin-2-ones. This heterocycle has an amide group present at the 1,2 position, with the carbonyl ("one") being present at the 2 position. The numbering system for the benzodiazepines is as shown.

▪ **PHYSICAL-CHEMICAL PROPERTIES.** Few distinctive properties of the benzodiazepines need concern us. The nitrogen at the 4 position is a basic, but only weakly basic, nitrogen. Salt formation at this position to give a water-soluble salt is usually not practiced, probably because of the weakness of this base (pK_a of protonated compound ~ 3.4). The nitrogen at the 1 position is weakly basic in the 3H-1,4-benzodiazepine and neutral in the amide 1,4-benzodiazepin-2-one structure.

▪ **METABOLISM.** Extensive data are available on the metabolism of the benzodiazepines. In many cases, the metabolism involves the additional substituents normally attached to the benzodiazepine nucleus. Metabolism of specific drugs will be discussed in the medicinal chemistry course. A common metabolic process that involves the 1,3-dihydro-2H-1,4-benzodiazepin-2-one nucleus is hydroxylation of the 3 position. This is seen with many of the anti-anxiety drugs.

TRICYCLIC HETEROCYCLES

▪ **NOMENCLATURE.** A wide variety of tricyclic heterocycles, some of which are of medicinal significance, might be presented. Three representative nuclei are shown in Figure 15-57: phenothiazine, dibenzazepine, and acridine. The nomenclature and numbering of these heterocycles are as shown. Note that the numbering system for each of these compounds is unique.

▪ **PHYSICAL-CHEMICAL PROPERTIES.** The phenothiazine nucleus contains a nitrogen that should be considered nearly neutral. Two aromatic rings attached to a nitrogen, each withdrawing electrons, reduce the basic property significantly. In most cases, this nitrogen will not form a salt with acid. The same reasoning holds for the nitrogen in 5H-dibenz[b,f]azepine. Acridine, although a weak base, can form salts with a strong acid.

An interesting physical property of the phenothiazine nucleus is that the molecule is not flat (Fig. 15-58). The shape of this molecule is thought to affect its biologic activity, and the amount of bend from planarity therefore may be important.

A characteristic of the acridine nucleus is the fact that the molecule possesses color. The nature of the color depends upon the substituents added to the three rings. The fact that a molecule possesses color indicates a highly conjugated molecule with alternating single and double bonds. With three conjugated rings, a yellow coloration is seen.

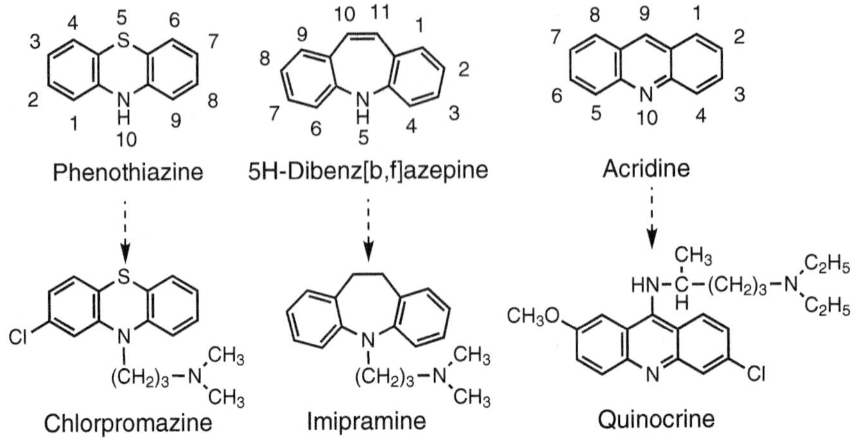

FIGURE 15-57. Structure of representative tricyclic heterocycles and examples of drugs containing these heterocycles.

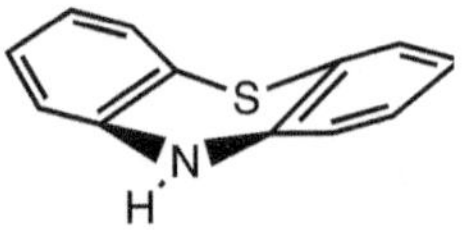

FIGURE 15-58. Conformational structure of phenothiazine.

■ **METABOLISM.** The characteristic metabolism found in all three of the tricyclic compounds is aromatic hydroxylation. Since the medicinally useful agents have substitution on these nuclei, the substitution will influence the site of hydroxylation.

An additional metabolism common to the phenothiazine nucleus is oxidation of the sulfur to the sulfoxide or sulfone. This reaction can be expected for any thioether and was discussed previously (see Fig. 8-6).

Case Study 15.1

Having taken an academic position at a prestigious pharmacy school after completing your postdoctoral education, you have quickly become one of the most highly respected teachers in the program. Students and colleagues alike appreciate your commitment to interdisciplinary collaboration and content integration, and the fact that you regularly reinforce the importance of medicinal chemistry in the rationale design and therapeutic use of drugs.

You have just started a series of lessons on diuretics and designed a structure-based therapeutic challenge for the class that involves the popular diuretic

(case study continues on page 131)

Case Study 15.1 (continued)

furosemide (Lasix). Specifically, you asked your students to identify two heterocyclic functional groups out of five choices that would be **bioisosteric** with
furosemide's oxygen-containing ring. To be bioisosteric, the replacement rings
must have essentially the same chemical properties as the original ring so that
the original biological activity could reasonably be assumed to be maintained.

Furosemide (Lasix)

Ring replacement candidates:

1   2   3   4   5

Having completed the in-class exercise, your students are now clamoring for
you to reveal the correct choices. Use the space below to write your answer key.

Case Study 15.2

You are a first year pharmacy student and are given the following case-based examination question in the course in organic functional groups. The professor wants to
test your ability to apply knowledge gained from the chapter on heterocycles.

PM, a 65-year-old Caucasian female, recently suffered an episode of uric
acid renal stones. PM has a history of asymptomatic hyperuricemia (plasma uric
acid ~9.5mg/dL). She developed severe diarrhea while on a vacation cruise,
which she said was brought on by something she ate. She knew enough to hy-
drate and did so with copious quantities of cranberry juice, which acidifies the
urine. However, PM developed nausea, vomiting, and intolerable flank pain,
which made her seek out the ship's doctor. Given PM's history of hyperuricemia
the doctor made a diagnosis of uric acid kidney stones and treated PM with
sodium bicarbonate (4 g stat, then 2 g every 4 hours not to exceed 16 g a day)
and told her to immediately stop drinking cranberry juice and switch to 2 to 3
L of water a day.

(case study continues on page 132)

Case Study 15.2 (continued)

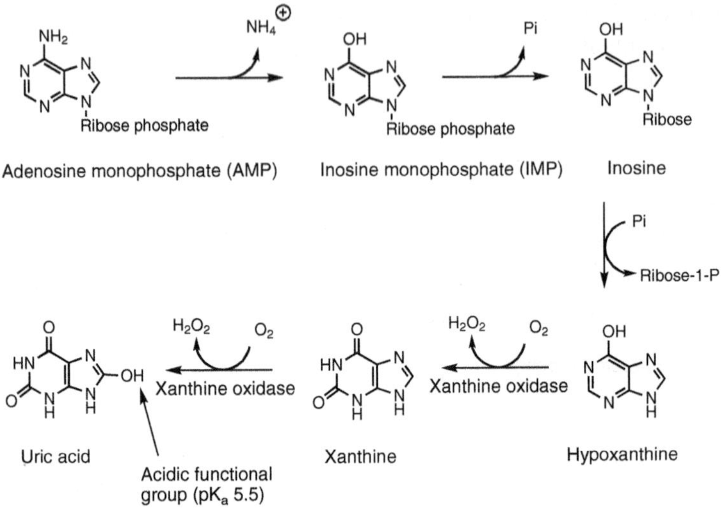

Metabolic degradation of the purine nucleotide adenosine monophosphate to uric acid.

Given that uric acid, the end product of purine metabolism, is a weak acid (pK_a = 5.5) formed by the action of xanthine oxidase on xanthine, and that PM's urinary pH is 5.0 answer the following questions:

1. Why did the doctor tell PM to immediately switch from cranberry juice to water?
2. What is the role of sodium bicarbonate in treating uric acid kidney stones?
3. Given that the most acidic functional group of uric acid and phenol are aromatic alcohols (phenolic hydroxy groups), can you explain the almost 1,000,000-fold difference in their pK_as (phenol pK_a = 11, uric acid pK_a = 5.5)?

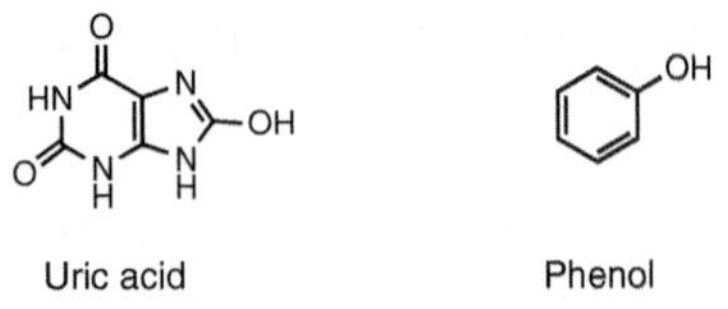

Uric acid   Phenol

Oligonucleotides and Nucleic Acids

16

By far the most important chemicals in all living cells are the nucleic acids deoxyribonucleic acid (DNA) and ribonucleic acid (RNA). These polymeric molecules are the sources of all information needed for the construction of a living organism and the production of the proteins that run the organism, respectively. DNA found in the nucleus of eukaryotic cells is a double-stranded polymer that makes up the genes of an organism. DNA uncoils into a "sense" strand of nucleic acid and an "antisense" strand. The "antisense" strand is transcribed into messenger RNA (mRNA), which has the same sequence as the "sense" strand of DNA. The mRNA leaves the nucleus and in the ribosome serves as the template defining the sequence for protein synthesis. Thus, DNA and its messenger RNA prescribe the construction of all of the proteins of the body that carry out the day-to-day function of the living organism.

■ **NOMENCLATURE.** The two nucleic acids, DNA and RNA, are made up of four heterocyclic bases: guanine, adenine, and cytosine (common to both DNA and RNA) and uracil or thymine, present in RNA and DNA, respectively (Fig. 16-1). As discussed in Chapter 15, guanine and adenine are purines, while cytosine, uracil, and thymine are pyrimidines. Two pentoses are present in the nucleic acids, and these pentoses are ribose or deoxyribose in RNA or DNA, respectively. When the pentoses are attached to the N-9 position of the purines or the N-1 position of the pyrimidines, the resulting product is named a *nucleoside*. The suffix "-side" indicates the presence of a sugar. Attachment of the sugar to the bases occurs at the 1′ position of the sugar. The linkage between the sugar and the heterocyclic base is through an acetal functional group. Finally, a phosphoric acid is added to the 5′ position of the pentose to give the *nucleotide*. The phosphate attachment to the sugar is considered an ester group. Nucleic acids result from the polymerization of nucleotides through ester formation of the 5′-phosphate to the 3′ alcohol of the pentose (Fig. 16-2). The continuous chain of pentose-3′,5′-diester is present as the backbone to this polymer.

An oligonucleotide is a short-chain polymer of nucleotides with the same three components: base, sugar, and phosphate ester. The significance of oligonucleotides is that they represent a new approach to drug therapy, and such agents are referred to as "antisense drugs." Such drugs are designed to block protein synthesis in diseases associated with an abnormal protein and overexpression of a normal protein. The antisense drug is designed to interact with mRNA through Watson-Crick base pairing, leading ultimately to the blockage or termination of the action of mRNA.

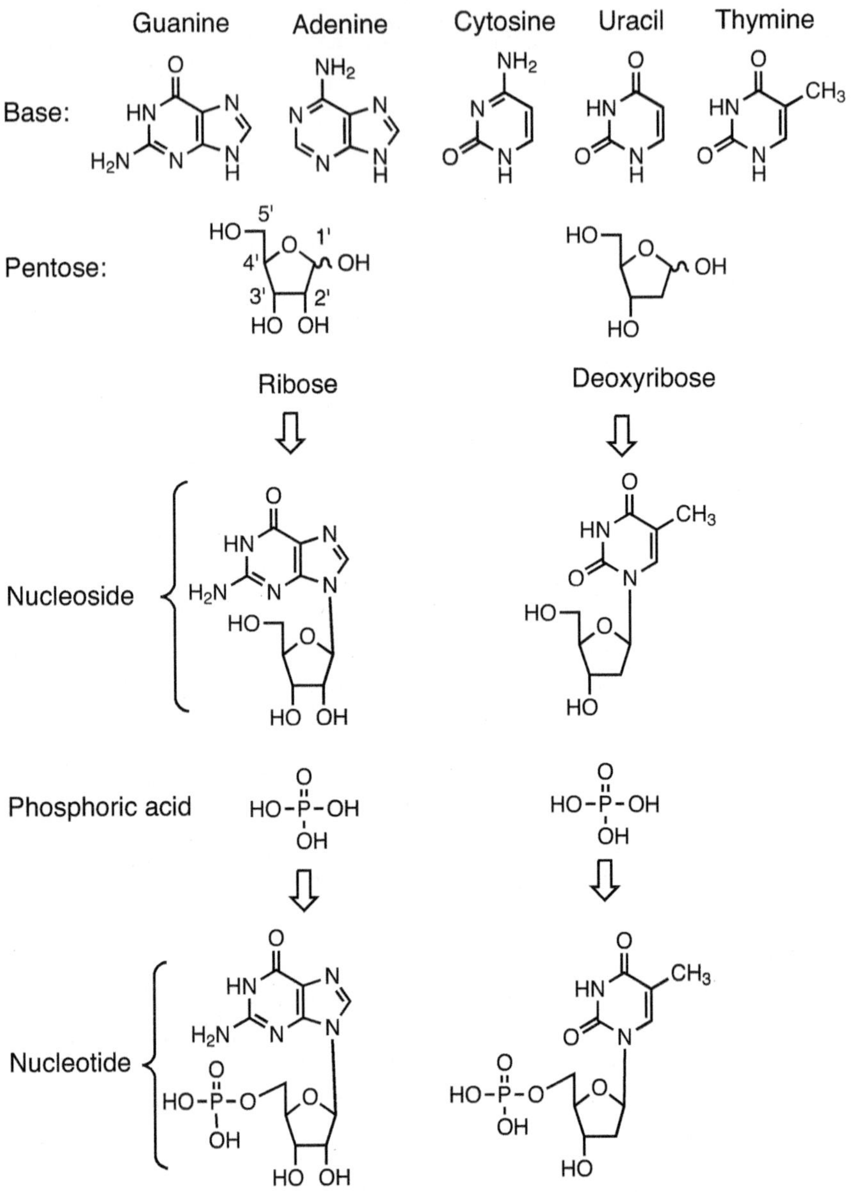

FIGURE 16-1. Structures of components of nucleotides.

The nomenclature used to identify the length of an oligonucleotide is to use an Arabic number corresponding to the number of nucleotides present, followed by "mer." Thus, the presence of 21 nucleotides would be to indicate the compound as a 21-mer oligonucleotide.

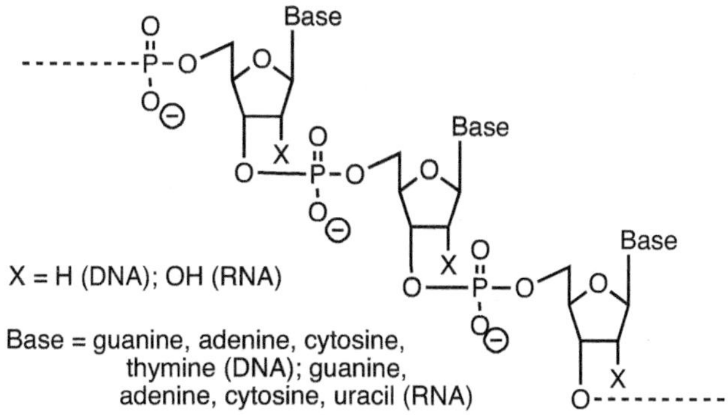

X = H (DNA); OH (RNA)

Base = guanine, adenine, cytosine,
thymine (DNA); guanine,
adenine, cytosine, uracil (RNA)

FIGURE 16-2. Structure of nucleic acids.

■ **PHYSICAL-CHEMICAL PROPERTIES.** The most significant physical-chemical properties possessed by oligonucleotides and nucleic acids are their hydrophilic-lipophilic properties and the ability of the various bases to recognize each other through hydrogen bonding. The backbone of the nucleotide diesters is hydrophilic in nature. At biologic pH, the phosphate diester is in an ionic state capable of ion-dipole bonding to water, and the pentose has hydrophilic character. The bases are usually considered hydrophobic in nature (Fig. 16-3).

The most unusual characteristic of nucleotides is the ability of the various bases to base pair through hydrogen bonding. The Watson-Crick model states that a guanine will base pair to a cytosine through three hydrogen bonds, while an adenine will base pair to thymine through two hydrogen bonds (Fig. 16-4). This base pairing in DNA thus results in the double helix, in which the ratio of guanine to cytosine is always 1 and the ratio of adenine to thymine is always 1. Because of the base pairing of the two strands of DNA, the hydrophobic bases are oriented to the

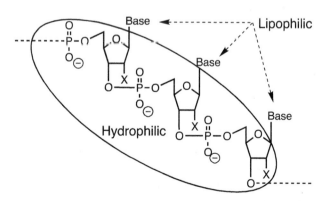

FIGURE 16-3. Lipophilic-hydrophilic portions of an oligonucleotide.

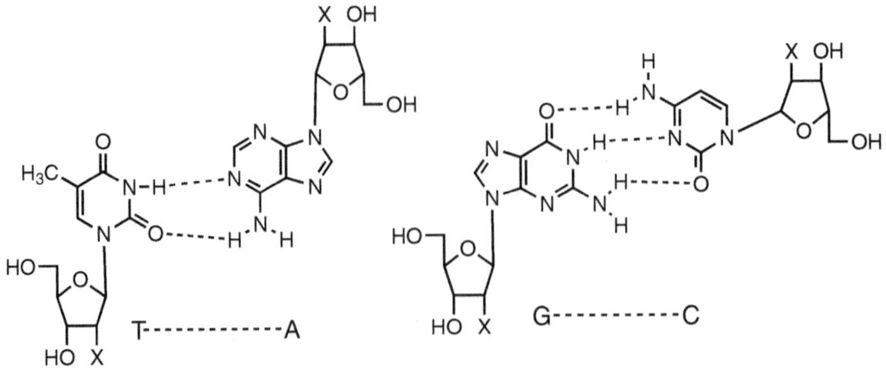

FIGURE 16-4. Base pairing of thymine (T) to adenine (A) and guanine (G) to cytosine (C).

inside of the double helix and the hydrophilic backbone is oriented to the outside of the helix.

Unlike DNA, RNA tends to exist as single strands with intermittent intramolecular base pairing, resulting in the formation of loops in the structure.

The design of oligonucleotide drugs (antisense drugs) is based upon the fact that deoxyribonucleotide analogs can base pair to complementary areas in mRNA and as a result can bind to a specific region of the mRNA to disrupt protein synthesis. This does require that one identify stretches of mRNA that are not base paired and that the chosen mRNA be associated with the aberrant protein.

Oligonucleotides present an in vitro stability problem in that they are prone to both acid- and base-catalyzed hydrolysis. The site most likely to undergo hydrolysis is at the phospho diester bond. The hydrolytic process leads to formation of oligonucleotide fragments, with a phosphate ester remaining at either the 3' or 5' position of the pentose. An interesting complication to the base-catalyzed hydrolysis of ribose-containing oligonucleotides has been seen. The ribose oligonucleotides are more likely to undergo base-catalyzed hydrolysis than their deoxyribose counterpart due to the participation of the 2'-OH in the hydrolysis reaction (Fig. 16-5).

■ **METABOLISM.** Common metabolism of oligonucleotides and nucleic acids is via nuclease enzymes. Such enzymes are common to most tissues of the body, and they can attack terminal phosphodiester bonds (exonucleases) or internal phosphodiester bonds (endonucleases) to break the backbone of the oligonucleotide or nucleic acid (Fig. 16-6). The design of nuclease-resistant drugs has turned to modification of the backbone of the oligonucleotide through changes in the structure of the phosphodiester or changes in the pentose. Examples of the former are phosphorothioates and methylphosphonates, while an example of the latter would be 2'-O-methylribonucleotide (Fig. 16-7). Such derivatives show increased stability toward cellular nucleases.

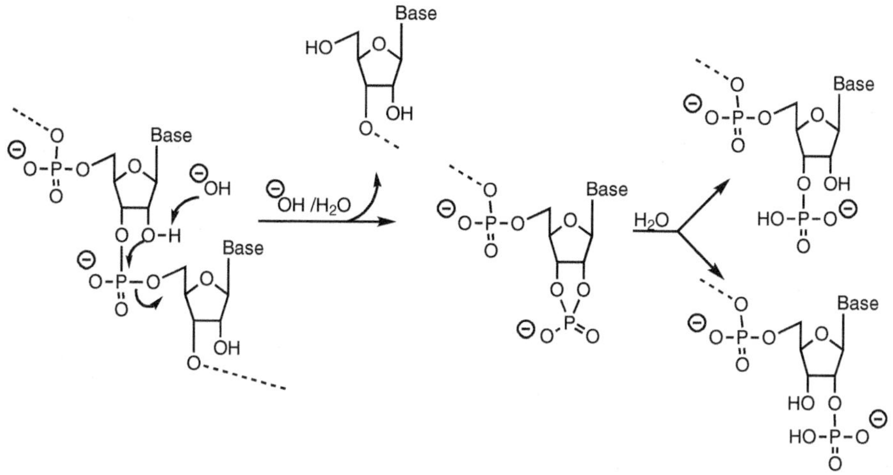

FIGURE 16-5. Base catalyzed hydrolysis of a ribose oligonucleotide.

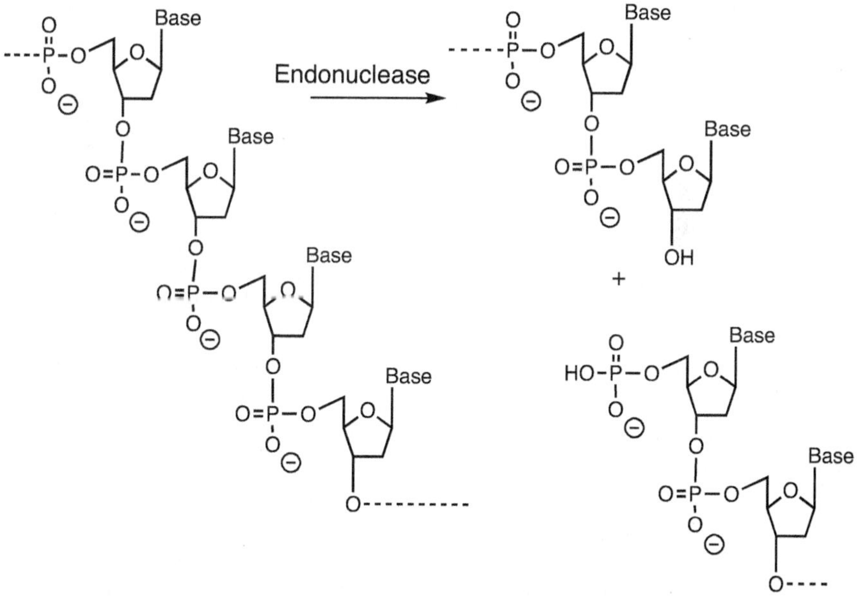

FIGURE 16-6. Metabolism of an oligonucleotide by endonuclease.

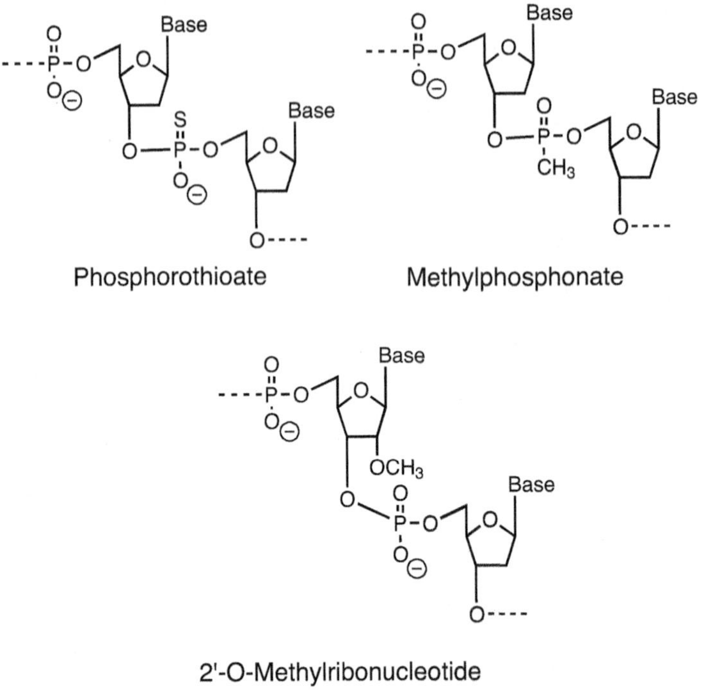

Phosphorothioate   Methylphosphonate

2'-O-Methylribonucleotide

FIGURE 16-7. Structural modification of oligonucleotides to protect against nuclease metabolism.

Case Study 16.1

You are the entrepreneur owner of **Drugs by Design** (*commonly known as D-by-D*) pharmacy, which specializes in compounding pharmaceuticals tailor-made for individual patients. It is National Pharmacy Week, and the **D-by-D** employees are volunteering at a local facility providing after-school services to economically disadvantaged youth. In addition to promoting the profession of pharmacy, your group is helping these young people with their math and science homework. One very bright teenager is taking biochemistry and learning about the nucleotides that comprise DNA and RNA. As a way of both helping her understand these essential structures and to show her how her understanding of nucleic acid biochemistry would serve her as a pharmacist, you challenge her with the following problem.

The DNA macromolecule is formed in the body by adding individual nucleotides (DNA "building blocks") one at a time to a growing DNA chain. The enzyme that catalyzes this reaction is called DNA polymerase. Compounds that inhibit DNA polymerase are potent anticancer agents. To fool DNA polymerase, the inhibitors must look a lot like the real DNA nucleotides. They are

(case study continues on page 139)

Case Study 16.1 (continued)

actually transported across cell membranes as nucleo*sides*, and then converted into nucleo*tides* inside the target cell. Only when they are in active nucleotide form can they be mistakenly incorporated into the DNA chain by the polymerase enzyme, and subsequently kill the cell.

The three fluorinated nucleic acid-based structures drawn below are actual drugs used in the treatment of cancer. Which one has the right chemistry to be a DNA polymerase inhibitor? What are the key chemical features of your chosen molecule that make it an appropriate choice? What's wrong with the remaining molecules? (**Hint:** The fluorine atom(s) in each structure are **not** the problem, as the polymerase initially mistakes it for the natural hydrogen atom. Look elsewhere on the structures to determine which is ... and which is not ... the polymerase inhibitor).

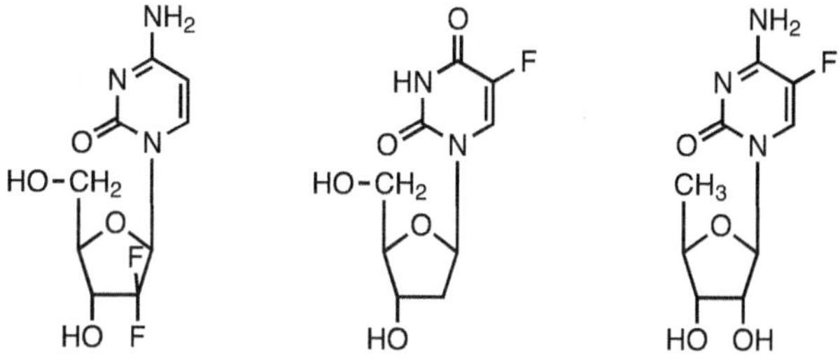

What answer are you hoping to get from this future pharmacist?

Case Study 16.2

You are working the night shift at the local inner city hospital pharmacy. You receive an order for AB, a 26-year-old female drug abuser who admitted to sharing unsterile needles with another addict for several years. AB tested positive for the human immunodeficiency virus (HIV) and has a CD4 lymphocyte count of 200 (a normal count ranges from 800 to 1,200). In addition she came to the hospital complaining of diarrhea, fever, and enlarged lymph glands and said she lost 22 lbs in the last 3 weeks. These symptoms indicated that she has the acquired immunodeficiency syndrome (AIDS). The physician's order calls for Combivir, a multidrug product that includes lamivudine and zidovudine (ZDV).

(case study continues on page 140)

Case Study 16.2 (continued)

The pharmacist on duty knows you are a first-year pharmacy student and takes this opportunity to reinforce some basics of organic functional groups. She draws the structures of these two drugs:

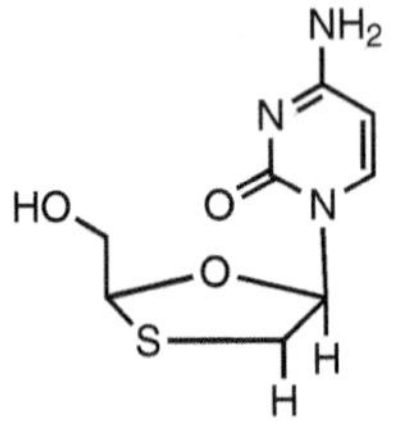

Lamivudine (3TC) 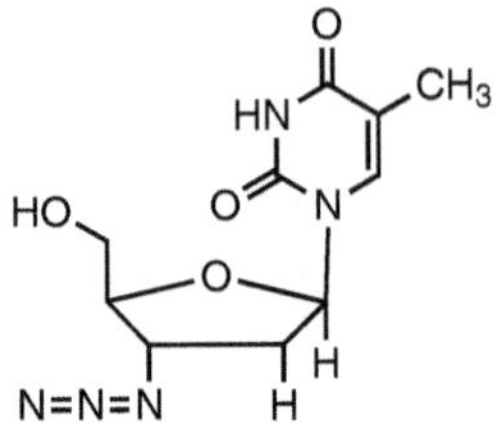   Zidovudine (ZDV)

She tells you the mechanism of action of these drugs is to inhibit viral nucleoside reverse transcriptase. Reverse transcriptase is a type of DNA polymerase that produces single-strand DNA from single-strand viral RNA. She then asks you to do the following:

1. Classify these structures as either nucleoside, nucleotide, or nucleic acid analogs. Explain your answer and can you identify which nucleoside, nucleotide, or nucleic acid these drugs mimic?
2. Explain how you think reverse transcriptase/DNA polymerase creates a DNA chain.
3. Identify the structural groups in each compound that explains why they can inhibit the viral reverse transcriptase.

Proteins

Another of the important macromolecules present in biologic systems are the polymers composed of amino acids and termed *proteins*. Derived from the Greek word *proteios* ("of the first order"), proteins have always occupied a significant niche in biochemistry instruction. From a pharmacologic standpoint, proteins have been recognized for their importance as enzymes catalyzing the reactions of the cell. They serve as key components of many, if not most, drug receptor sites. They have an important role in drug transport, and they have biologic activity as hormones. These naturally occurring materials may be relatively small molecules consisting of a few amino acids (Fig. 17-1) to extremely large-molecular-weight compounds made up of hundreds of amino acids. In the past, medicinal chemistry coverage of proteins has been limited because only a few protein drugs were available and the complexity of their synthesis, purification, chemistry, and administration made an in-depth discussion difficult and unproductive. With the recent discoveries in recombinant DNA technology, methods in hybridoma technology, automated protein synthesis, and newer methods of drug delivery, however, proteinaceous drugs are now not only possible but in fact have begun to appear on the market, with the expectation that scores of additional drugs will appear in the near future. As a result it is extremely important to be familiar with the basic chemical features of protein stability in vitro as well as potential protein metabolism.

■ **NOMENCLATURE.** Naturally occurring proteins are made up of 20 amino acids. These 20 amino acids are linked through amide bonds into a polymeric structure called a polypeptide or the protein. The arrangement of the amino acids within the protein is determined by the organism's DNA structure, as translated by messenger RNA (mRNA). The amino acids making up the protein may be neutral, acidic, or basic amino acids (Table 17-1).

The arrangement of amino acids in the protein gives the primary structure of the protein. The three-dimensional structure of a protein (i.e., how it is arranged in space) will define the protein's secondary, tertiary, or quaternary structure. The spatial arrangements of a protein are discussed in detail in *Foye's Principles of Medicinal Chemistry*, Chapter 7. The presentation of a protein structure may appear in various forms, examples of which are shown in Figure 17-1. Commonly, the structure is shown using the abbreviations for the various amino acids, since the other representations are difficult to interpret and to draw.

■ **PHYSICAL-CHEMICAL PROPERTIES.** Although several unique physical-chemical properties are associated with proteins, some properties are predictable based

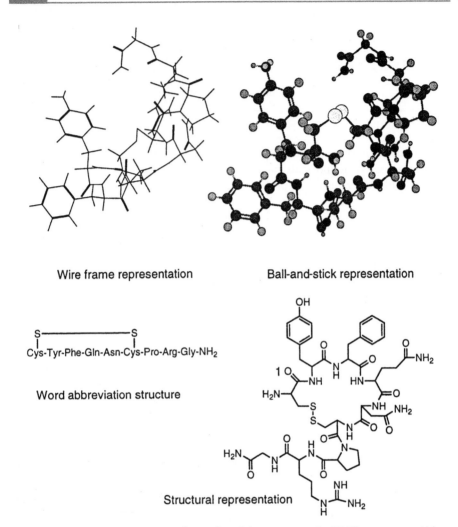

Wire frame representation   Ball-and-stick representation

Word abbreviation structure

Structural representation

FIGURE 17-1. Various representations of arginine vasopressin (AVP), a nonapeptide.

upon the properties of the monomers that make up the polymeric macromolecules. The individual units that constitute the structure of proteins are the 20 amino acids, 19 of which are chiral molecules possessing the L-configuration. Amino acids are characteristically hydrophilic; this same property is found in proteins. Because of this hydrophilic nature, proteins tend to show poor penetration through lipophilic membranes, such as the intestinal lining, cell membranes, and blood-brain barrier.

Chemical instability of proteins follows a pattern related to the functionality of the individual amino acids present in the protein. The general types of chemical reactions seen in proteins consist of oxidation-reduction, deamidation, hydrolysis, and racemization reactions.

Table 17-1. STRUCTURES OF NATURAL AMINO ACIDS

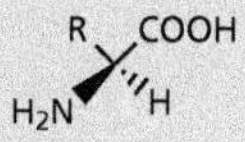

$$R \underset{H_2N}{\overset{COOH}{\diagup}} H$$

AMINO ACID	ABBREVIATION	STRUCTURE R=
Neutral:		
Glycine	Gly, G	$H-$
Alanine	Ala, A	H_3C-
Isoleucine	Ile, I	$C_2H_5-\overset{CH_3}{\underset{\|}{C}H}-$
Leucine	Leu, L	$H_3C-\overset{CH_3}{\underset{\|}{C}H}-CH_2-$
Valine	Val, V	$H_3C-\overset{CH_3}{\underset{\|}{C}H}-$
Cysteine	Cys, C	$HS-CH_2-$
Methionine	Met, M	$H_3C-S-CH_2-CH_2-$
Serine	Ser, S	$HO-CH_2-$
Threonine	Thr, T	$H_3C-\underset{\underset{OH}{\|}}{C}H-$
Asparagine	Asn, N	$H_2N-\overset{O}{\overset{\|}{C}}-CH_2-$
Glutamine	Gln, Q	$H_2N-\overset{O}{\overset{\|}{C}}-(CH_2)_2-$
Phenylalanine	Phe, F	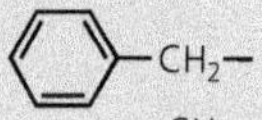 $\langle phenyl \rangle-CH_2-$
Tryptophan	Trp, W	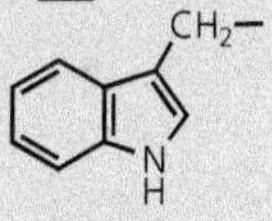 indole$-CH_2-$
Proline	Pro, P	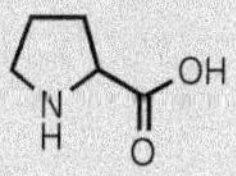 proline ring
Acidic:		
Aspartic acid	Asp, D	$HO-\overset{O}{\overset{\|}{C}}-CH_2-$
Glutamic acid	Glu, E	$HO-\overset{O}{\overset{\|}{C}}-(CH_2)_2-$
Tyrosine	Tyr, Y	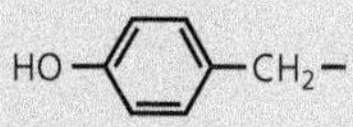 $HO-\langle phenyl \rangle-CH_2-$
Basic:		
Arginine	Arg, R	$H_2N-\overset{NH}{\overset{\|}{C}}-\overset{H}{\underset{}{N}}-(CH_2)_3-$
Lysine	Lys, K	$H_2N-(CH_2)_4-$
Histidine	His, H	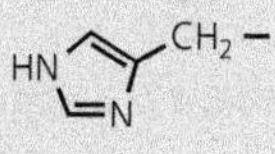 imidazole$-CH_2-$

Oxidation Reactions.   The amino acids most prone to oxidation reactions consist of methionine (Met), cysteine (Cys), histidine (His), tryptophan (Try), and tyrosine (Tyr). The amino acid methionine contains a thioether functional group (Fig. 17-2). This unit is readily oxidized by mild oxidizing agents, such as hydrogen peroxide, as well as oxygen in the air, and represents a potential problem for storage of proteins.

The amino acid cysteine contains the thiol functional group, which is also readily oxidized to any of a number of oxidation states, depending on the strength of the oxidizing agent. Potentially the simplest oxidation may be the conversion of the thiol to a disulfide (cystine), a reaction that occurs in the presence of oxygen and metal ions (Fig. 17-3). The reverse of this reaction (i.e., the reduction of a disulfide linkage of cystine) may also occur readily during protein isolation and purification. Since intramolecular and intermolecular disulfide bonds are common in proteins, a reduction of the disulfide bond will result in significant changes in the physical-chemical properties of the protein as well as the biologic activity of the protein. The disulfide bond forces the protein to adopt a specific shape, and thus breaking this bond allows the molecule to "unfold" and take on a new shape, which results in totally different properties. Disulfide bonds are quite common in biologically active proteins including molecules such as vasopressin (see Fig. 17-1), somatostatin, oxytocin, parathyroid hormone, and insulin.

The oxidation of histidine, tryptophan, and tyrosine has been reported to occur with a variety of oxidizing agents. In those cases in which oxidation occurs, it is thought that the aromatic ring is cleaved, but structures of the breakdown products have not been characterized. With histidine and tryptophan, it is postulated that the products of oxidation are aspartic acid and N-formyl kynurenine, respectively (Fig. 17-4).

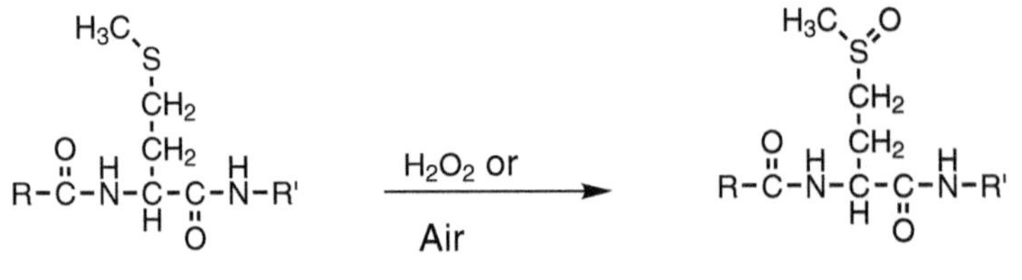

FIGURE 17-2. Oxidation of methionine.

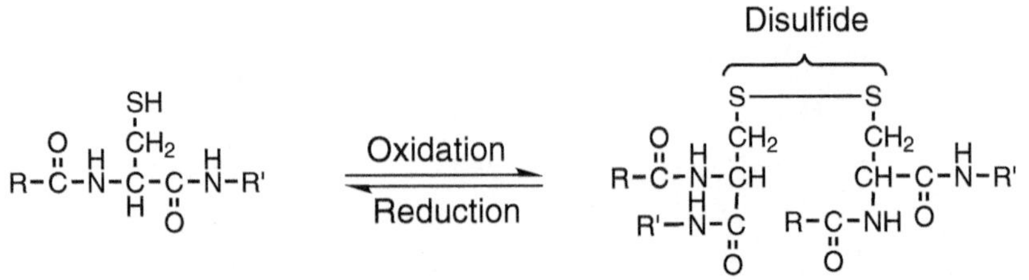

FIGURE 17-3. Oxidation of cysteine, reduction of cystine.

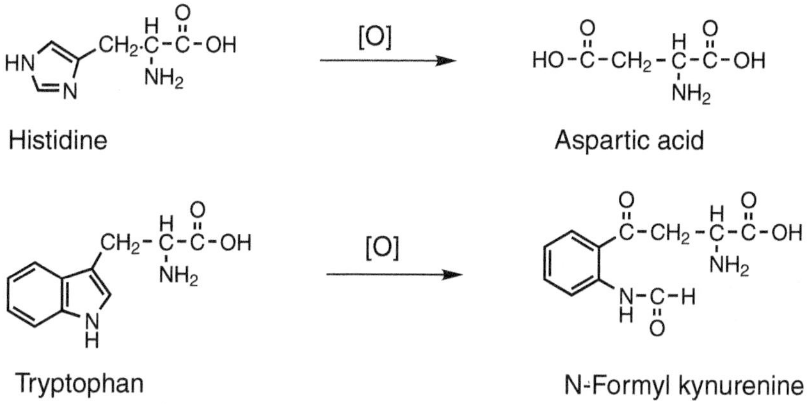

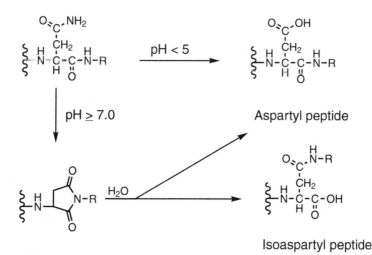

FIGURE 17-4. Oxidation of histidine and tryptophan.

Deamidation Reactions. A common in vitro reaction of asparagine (Asn) and possibly of glutamine (Gln) is the hydrolysis of the side chain amide. This reaction has been investigated extensively for asparagine, with the nature of the products being influenced by the pH of the medium. If the pH is strongly acidic, a simple hydrolysis occurs, resulting in formation of the aspartyl peptide (Fig. 17-5). When the protein is stored at neutral or alkaline pH, not only is the aspartyl peptide produced but in addition the isoaspartyl peptide can be isolated. This reaction has been shown to proceed through a cyclic imide intermediate that opens readily to give the two possible products (see Fig. 17-5). These changes can be expected to have a profound effect on the physical-chemical properties and the biologic activity of the modified protein.

FIGURE 17-5. Deamidation of asparagine-containing protein at acidic or basic pH.

A similar process can be invoked for hydrolysis of the glutamine side chain, but at present there is little supportive chemical evidence to suggest that this reaction is a serious problem in vitro.

Hydrolysis Reaction. Hydrolysis of peptide bonds in a protein generally does not occur. The typical amide bond is relatively stable with one exception. An aspartate (Asp) residue in the protein greatly increases the potential for hydrolysis of the peptide at the N-terminal and/or C-terminal position of this amino acid at acidic pH. The presence of a side chain carboxyl is important since this group assists the hydrolysis reaction, as shown in Figure 17-6. The hydrolysis obviously results in destruction of the protein.

Racemization Reaction. Nineteen of the 20 amino acids contain a chiral center that in theory could be racemized under basic conditions to the D-**enantiomer**, thus resulting in a protein with large differences in physical-chemical properties and biologic activities. Most amino acids appear to be relatively stable to racemization, although some evidence suggests that aspartate residues may racemize through a cyclic imide (Fig. 17-7). The formation of the cyclic imide increases the ease of proton removal at the asymmetric carbon, which upon reprotonation leads to formation of both isomers. Presumably resonance stabilization of the α-carbanion in the imide plays an important role in the racemization reaction.

Conformational Changes. A unique property found in proteins, but not commonly found in the low-molecular-weight compounds previously dealt with, is the high degree of intramolecular and intermolecular bonding that occurs in proteins. The amide functional groups found in protein can act as both a hydrogen donor and a hydrogen acceptor, leading to hydrogen bonding. If the hydrogen

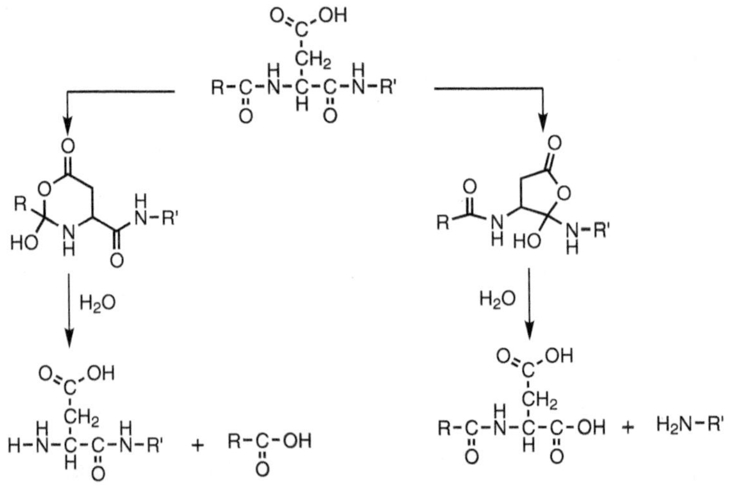

FIGURE 17-6. Hydrolysis of aspartate-containing protein.

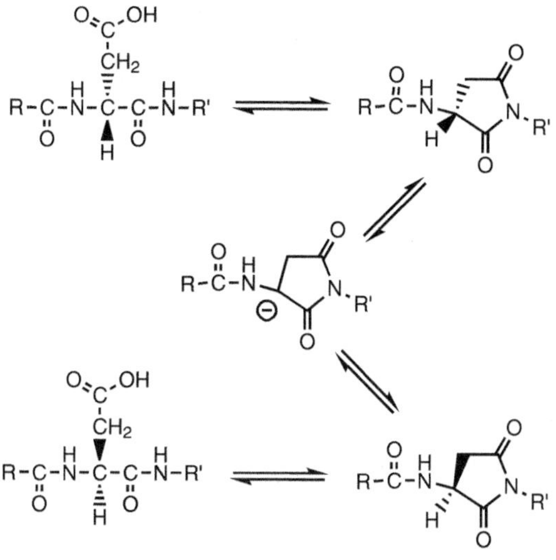

FIGURE 17-7. Racemization of the aspartate residue in proteins.

bonding occurs intramolecularly between the first and fourth peptide bond, the α-helix conformation results (Fig. 17-8), but if the hydrogen bonding occurs intermolecularly (or intramolecularly with a distant portion of the same protein), the β-sheet conformation is found (Fig. 17-9). The conformation of the protein resulting from the spatial arrangement and interactions due to nearby amino acids is referred to as the **secondary** structure of the protein. This secondary structure for the protein leads to a great deal of rigidity, but a rigidity that can be broken by temperature variations, changes in pH, or the presence of organic solvents. Molecules that are coiled or tightly packed due to hydrogen bonding have different physical-chemical and biologic properties than their nonbonded form. Another phenomenon seen with proteins is that they fold in such a way that the hydrophobic groups are buried in the interior of the polypeptide, while the hydrophilic groups are on the surface of the protein. The protein becomes globular in structure. The globular

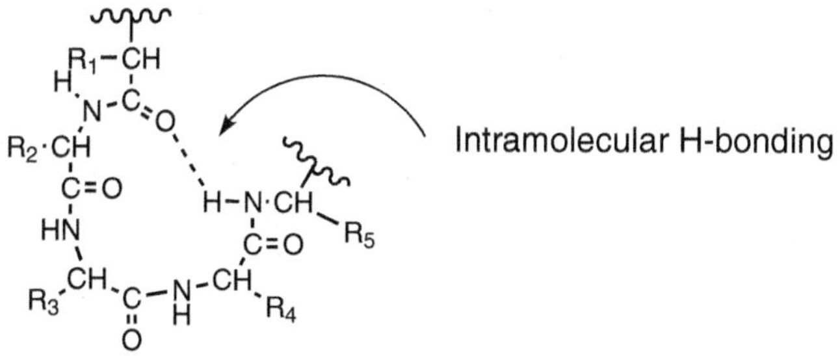

FIGURE 17-8. H-bonding resulting in an α-helix protein structure.

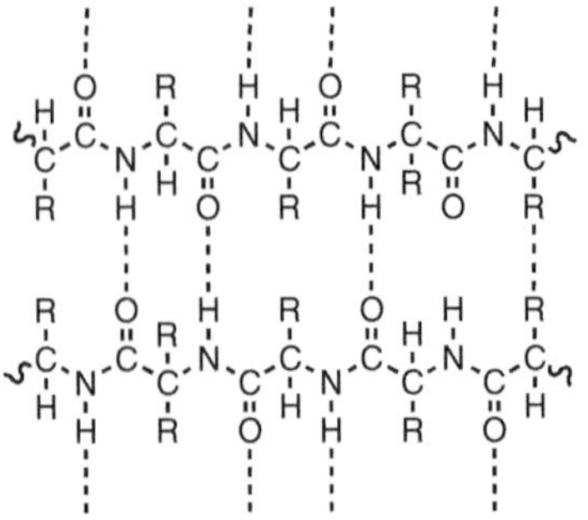

FIGURE 17-9. H-bonding resulting in a β-sheet protein structure.

long-distance conformation of a protein is referred to as the **tertiary** structure. Water binds readily to the protein, while van der Waals bonding occurs in the interior. This conformation of a protein confers specific physical-chemical and biologic activity to the protein. Once again, the globular conformation of the protein can be destroyed by temperature, pH, and solvent changes. The secondary and tertiary structures of the molecule are changed and the protein is said to be **denatured**. Unlike low-molecular-weight compounds, the polymeric proteins must be protected from drastic changes in temperature during storage, pH of the surrounding medium, and the presence of organic solvents.

■ **METABOLISM.** A wide variety of metabolic reactions have been reported to occur in proteins, complicated to some extent by the fact that these reactions may be highly specific for a particular amino acid or for a certain dipeptide pattern. The types of metabolic reactions anticipated are oxidation-reduction reactions and hydrolysis reactions.

Oxidation Reductions. Similar to the oxidation reactions seen in vitro, it would be expected that methionine and cysteine would experience metabolic oxidation to give a sulfoxide and a disulfide, respectively (see Figs. 17-2 and 17-3). The resulting changes would be expected to produce proteins with physical-chemical properties and biologic activity quite different from those seen in the native protein. The oxidation of a cysteine to the disulfide or the reduction of a disulfide to the thiol of a cysteine changes the primary structure of a protein. For example, proteins containing disulfide bonds commonly have a cyclic structure (Fig. 17-10). If this bond is reduced, the cysteines, which were connected to each other (cystine), now may be separated by a great distance in the linear chain. The shape of the protein has undergone a drastic change and will lose whatever biologic activity it possessed. To return activity to a reduced protein requires oxidation of the thiol to the disulfide, and if several cysteines are present in the protein, an incorrect pairing may occur, leading to non-native protein with the incorrect three-dimensional structure.

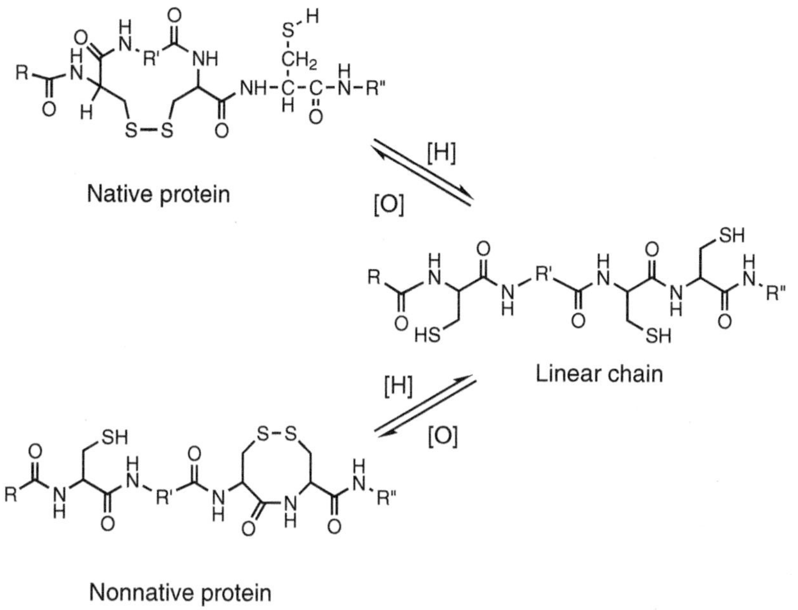

FIGURE 17-10. Reduction of the disulfide bond in a protein and oxidation of the thiol to the disulfide.

Hydrolysis of Peptides. The breakdown of proteins under the influence of hydrolyzing enzymes can occur throughout the body. Intestinal fluids contain a variety of peptidases, such as trypsin, chymotrypsin, elastase, and carboxypeptidase. Commonly found in the small intestine, these peptidases can completely degrade protein within a few minutes. But additionally, peptidases or their precursors may be found in the blood, in nerve synaptic regions, in the skin, and in fact in most fluids and tissues of the body. Therefore, the rapid metabolism of peptides can be expected, with the resulting termination of biologic activity.

A variety of aminopeptidases, carboxypeptidases, and deamidases attack and hydrolyze amide bonds. These enzymes may be highly selective for specific amino acids or combinations of amino acids. Table 17-2 lists the selectivity for several common enzymes. In general, aminopeptidase cleaves proteins starting at the N-terminal amino acid, carboxypeptidase cleaves amino acids from the C-terminal end of the peptide, and deamidases hydrolyze simple unsubstituted amides. As an example of the metabolism of a natural protein, Figure 17-11 outlines the metabolism of arginine vasopressin in intestinal juice, while Figure 17-12 indicates the metabolic fate of arginine vasopressin in brain synapses.

Table 17-2. PROTEIN HYDROLYZING ENZYMES

ENZYME	SELECTIVITY
Trypsin	Cleaves on carboxyl side of lysine and arginine
Thrombin	Cleaves arginine and glycine
Chymotrypsin	Cleaves on carboxyl side of aromatic amino acids (Tyr, Trp, Phe) and methionine
Pepsin	Cleaves tyrosine, tryptophan, and phenylalanine
Carboxypeptidase A	Cleaves carboxy-terminal peptides (faster for aromatics and bulky aliphatic amino acids)
Carboxypeptidase B	Cleaves arginine and lysine
Elastase	Cleaves amide bonds of small and uncharged amino acids

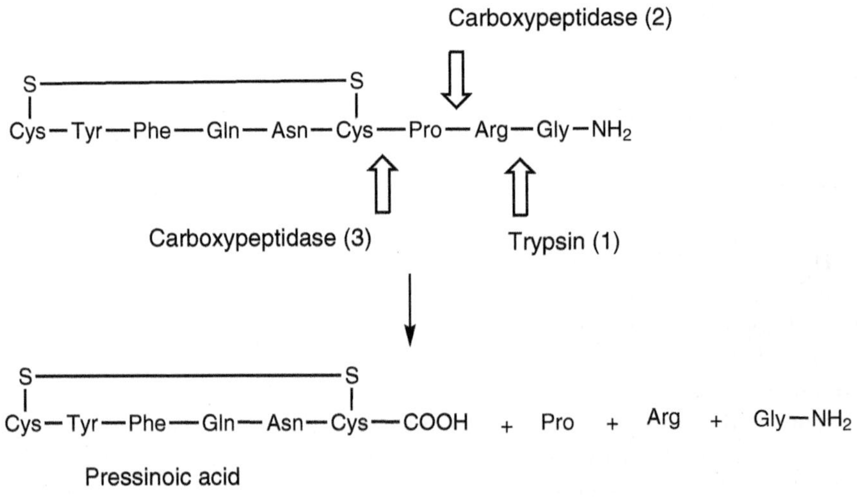

Carboxypeptidase (2)

S——————————————S
| |
Cys—Tyr—Phe—Gln—Asn—Cys—Pro—Arg—Gly—NH₂

Carboxypeptidase (3)   Trypsin (1)

S————————————S
| |
Cys—Tyr—Phe—Gln—Asn—Cys—COOH   +   Pro   +   Arg   +   Gly—NH₂

Pressinoic acid

FIGURE 17-11. Intestinal metabolism of arginine vasopressin.

S——————————————S
| |
Cys—Tyr—Phe—Gln—Asn—Cys—Pro—Arg—Gly—NH₂

1   2   3   4

N-Terminus aminopeptidase

HOOC—Cys—S—S
           |
    H₂N—Asn—Cys—Pro—Arg—Gly—NH₂   +   Tyr   +   Phe   +   Gln

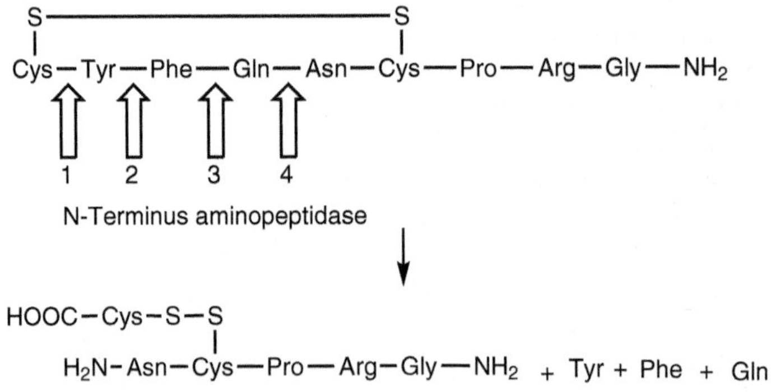

FIGURE 17-12. Brain synaptic metabolism of arginine vasopressin.

Case Study 17.1

As a conscientious senior pharmacy student interested in global health, and particularly passionate about providing care to underserved populations, you have elected an advanced practice rotation in the rural regions of Haiti. It's Friday afternoon, and you are working with your team in a remote Haitian village. You have just made an IV solution of oxytocin (a protein used to induce labor) that you've placed in a cold box set at 8°C (46°F). The team physician intends to use this IV on Monday morning if a pregnant patient who is 5 days past her due date has not delivered on her own.

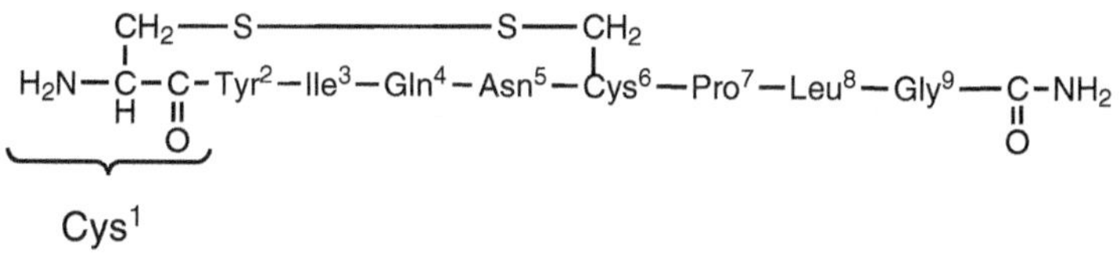

Oxytocin

Late Friday night a tropical storm blows through the area and, on Monday morning, you find that the power to the cold box was lost. It's not clear how long the oxytocin solution was stored outside the approved temperature range (36–77°F), but weekend highs were close to 100°F. The oxytocin solution appears a bit hazy and the physician tells you to discard it. However, since he just read an interesting article by A. Hawe et al. on oxytocin stability in the April 3, 2009 issue of *Pharmaceutical Research*, he first wants to test your knowledge of peptide degradation. He tells you two things:

1. Some of the oxytocin in the warm solution is most probably existing as a dimer (accounting for the haziness).
2. The oxytocin solution may contain ammonia (NH_3) as a by-product of degradation.

Based on these two clues, he asks you to predict at least one structure that could be found in the decomposed oxytocin solution. How do you respond?

Case Study 17.2

You made vacation plans with one of your friends almost a year ago, and the departure date is coming soon. Unfortunately, you are concerned that your vacation plans might be cancelled because your friend has been complaining of feeling sick for the last 3 weeks. When describing her symptoms to you, she say

(case study continues on page 152)

Case Study 17.2 (continued)

she has had pain in the upper right part of her abdomen, is extremely lethargic, and hardly has any appetite. When her skin and eyes started to take on a yellow color, her mother took her to the doctor. She had blood tests done and her alanine aminotransferase and aspartate aminotransferase enzyme plasma levels were above the upper limit of normal. You know that she has been an injection-drug user in the past, but has received drug abuse treatment and has been drug free for the last 6 months. When she goes back to the doctor, she is diagnosed with Hepatitis C and prescribed the drug Pegasys (Peg-interferon alfa-2a). Fortunately, this diagnosis won't disrupt your vacation plans; however, your friend complains that the medication must be administered subcutaneously, that her injection sites often hurt, and it is psychologically difficult for her to use needles anymore. As a pharmacy student, she asks you why she cannot take her medication orally. What is your answer for her?

Since you are a P-1 pharmacy student you are unfamiliar with Peg-interferon alfa-2a, so you look up the structure and discover that it is a high molecular weight branched monomethoxy polyethylene glycol conjugate of interferon alfa-2a.

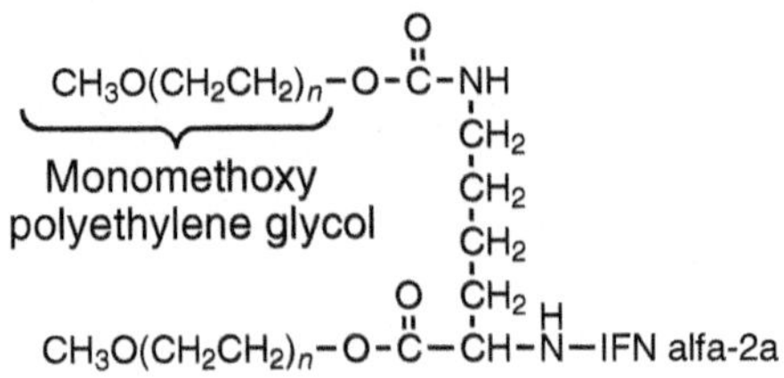

$$CH_3O(CH_2CH_2)_n{-}O{-}\overset{\displaystyle O}{\overset{\|}{C}}{-}NH$$

Monomethoxy
polyethylene glycol

$$\begin{array}{l} CH_2 \\ CH_2 \\ CH_2 \\ CH_2 \end{array}$$

$$CH_3O(CH_2CH_2)_n{-}O{-}\overset{\displaystyle O}{\overset{\|}{C}}{-}CH{-}\overset{\displaystyle H}{\underset{}{N}}{-}IFN\ alfa\text{-}2a$$

Peg-interferon alfa-2a ($n = 420\text{–}510$)

Predicting Water Solubility

THE ROLE OF CHEMICAL BONDING BETWEEN DISSIMILAR ORGANIC FUNCTIONAL GROUPS

We have now reviewed the major functional groups that might be expected in drug molecules. It will soon become obvious to you that the majority of the drugs discussed are not simple monofunctional molecules but instead are polyfunctional molecules. Most drugs will be found to contain two, three, four, or more of the organic functional groups within a single chemical entity, each of which contributes to the overall biologic activity, pharmacokinetic properties, and/or physical-chemical properties. To appreciate the role played by the various functional groups within the complex drug molecule it is necessary to recognize that each group may exhibit inter- and intramolecular bonding to other functional groups that could and does influence such factors as absorption, distribution, metabolism, excretion, receptor-binding affinity, and solubility of the drug. In general, the chemical properties, namely in vitro stability and in vivo stability, can be predicted based upon single group reactivity and each functional group can be treated independent of the other functional groups present. However, the reader should recognize that **intramolecular bonding** can influence metabolism and in vitro (shelf) stability. Numerous examples exist where intramolecular and intermolecular bonding does effect the solubility properties of mixed functional molecules.

If we consider the important physical property of water solubility, we find that polyfunctional molecules often behave differently than monofunctional molecules. A simple summation of the water-solubilizing properties of each functional group usually does not lead to a successful prediction of water solubility for the more complex systems. With a single functional group, there is no possibility of intramolecular bonding, that is, bonding within the molecule, because no other functional group is present. On the other hand, with polyfunctional molecules, intramolecular bonding may become a significant bonding interaction.

With the individual functional groups, intermolecular bonding is a factor in the solubilizing potential of the groups. For example, an alcohol functional group in a molecule such as hexanol binds to a second molecule of hexanol through dipole-dipole bonding. This bonding must be broken in order to dissolve the hexanol in water. When one states that an alcohol functional group solubilizes approximately six carbon atoms, one has already considered the intermolecular bonding of this type. But what about the polyfunctional molecules? The intermolecular bonding between like functional groups can still occur, but now new types of bonding are possible.

Bonding may occur between dissimilar functional groups through both an intermolecular and intramolecular type, and this bonding may be quite strong. In order for a molecule to dissolve in water, the intramolecular and intermolecular bonding must first be broken so that the water molecules can bond to the functional groups.

Intramolecular Bonding

One of the most significant examples of a mixed functional group intramolecular bond is seen with α-amino acids. Due to the basicity of an amine and the acidic character of the carboxylic acid, α-amino acids can exist in a zwitterion (internal salt) form through ion-ion bonding. The intramolecular bond destroys the ability of the individual groups to bond to water leading to reduced water solubility. The α-amino acids

also demonstrates a critical factor essential to intramolecular bonding, and that is that the functional groups must be in close proximity to each other (commonly within two to four carbon atoms of each other or within a molecule flexible enough to bring the two units into close proximity). With dipole-dipole or dipole-ion intramolecular bonding between mixed functional groups a pseudo five to seven member arrangement can be drawn (Fig. 18.1, **A–D**). Larger or smaller arrangements of bonding atoms are less favored. This arrangement and the types of functional groups involved are shown in Figure 18.1. The functional groups capable of donating a hydrogen for dipole-dipole bonds have been discussed individually in the appropriate chapters and include alcohols, phenols, the enol of a ketone, carboxylic acids and to a lesser but still potentially significant extent 1° and 2° amines. The functional groups which can dipole-dipole bond through acceptance of an hydrogen due to their electron-rich environment include the oxygen atom of alcohols, phenols, ethers, ketones and aldehydes, carboxylic acids, and the nitrogen atom of unionized 1°, 2° and 3° amines. It should be noted that several functional groups are capable of both donation of hydrogen as well as acceptance of a hydrogen through an electron-rich environment (Fig. 18.1, **A**). Also shown in Figure 18.1 (**D**) that ion-dipole bonding between mixed functional groups can occur with ionized carboxylates and hydrogen-donor functional groups, while protonated amines form ion-dipole bonds with electron-rich regions in the dipoles of alcohols, phenols, ethers, ketones and aldehydes, and carboxylic acids.

Examples of several drugs in which intramolecular bonding influences physical-chemical properties of these drugs are shown in Figure 18.2.

Intermolecular Bonding

In the individual functional group chapters, consideration was given to the ability of a functional group to bond to water or to bond to the same group in a second molecule. This property was used to predict water solubility and boiling

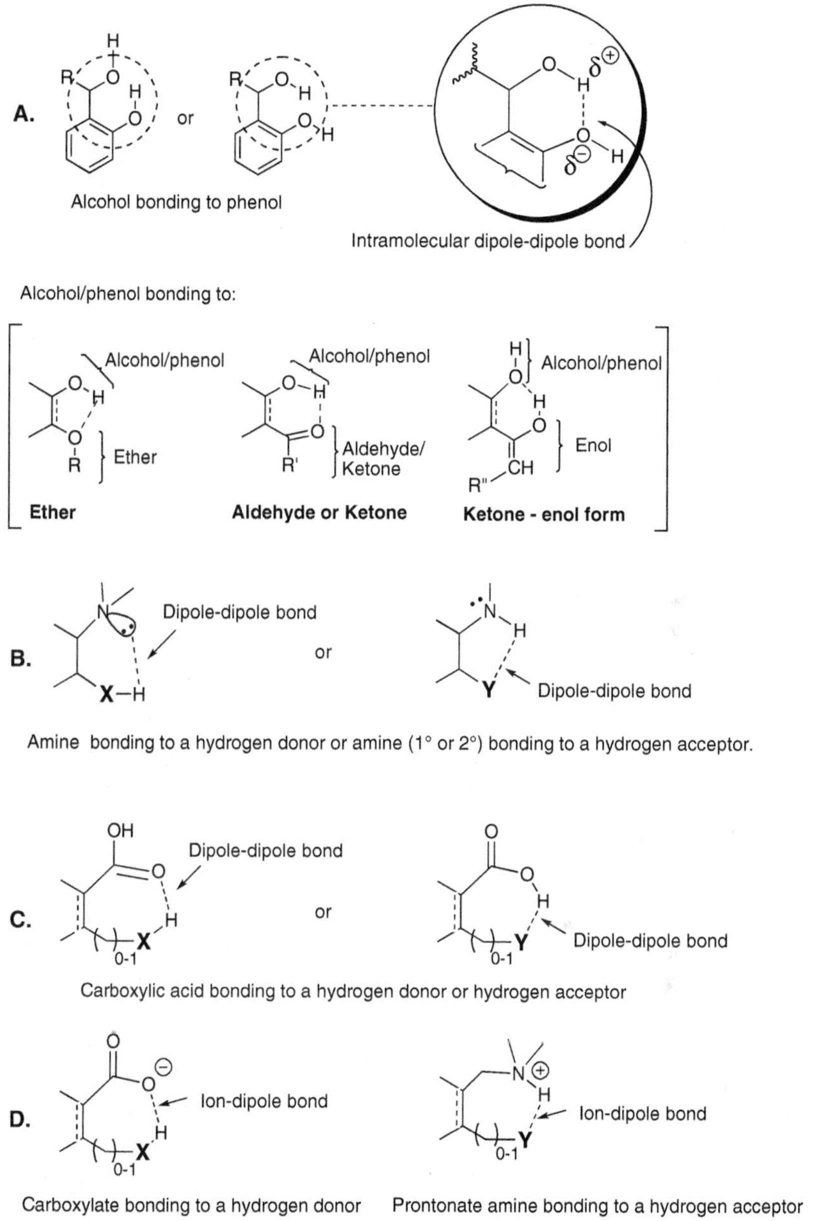

A.

Alcohol bonding to phenol

Intramolecular dipole-dipole bond

Alcohol/phenol bonding to:

Ether   **Aldehyde or Ketone**   **Ketone - enol form**

B.

Amine bonding to a hydrogen donor or amine (1° or 2°) bonding to a hydrogen acceptor.

C.

Carboxylic acid bonding to a hydrogen donor or hydrogen acceptor

D.

Carboxylate bonding to a hydrogen donor   Prontonate amine bonding to a hydrogen acceptor

X = electronegative atom (oxygen or nitrogen) capable of donating an attached hydrogen
  (i.e., the hydrogen of an alcohol, phenol, enol, or 1° or 2° amine).
Y = electronegative atom (oxygen or nitrogen) capable of accepting an hydrogen (i.e., the oxygen of
  an alcohol, phenol, enol, ether, carbonyl of a ketone or aldehyde, and the nitrogen of an amine).

FIGURE 18-1. Examples of intramolecular bonding between dissimilar
organic functional groups.

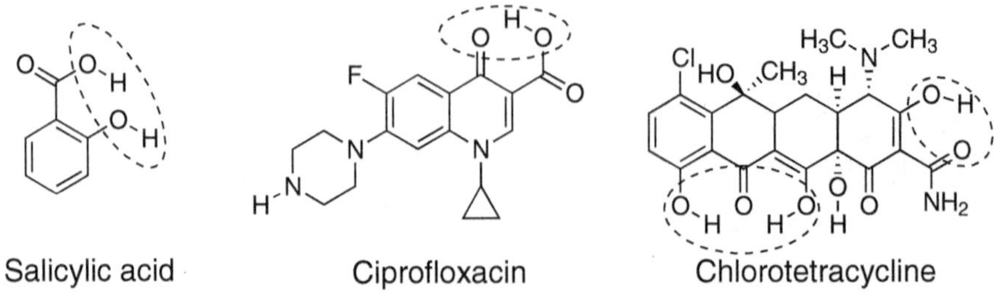

Salicylic acid   Ciprofloxacin   Chlorotetracycline

FIGURE 18-2. Examples of drugs where intramolecular bonding between dissimilar functional groups effects physical-chemical and pharmacodynamic properties of the drug.

points, respectively. Whether the functional group bonds to its counterpart in a second molecule or to a different functional in the second molecule the process is the same as the intramolecular process discussed above. The only difference is that intramolecular bonding tends to be stronger than intermolecular bonding. Thus, the same discussion and figure (Fig. 18-1) can represent mixed functional group intermolecular bonding. In this case the two functional groups are not brought together through covalent bonds, but instead through space. Two molecules and their respective functional groups must come close to each other and electron-rich regions need to be attracted to electron-deficient regions found in dipoles or ions for bonding to occur. Thus, alcohols, phenols, aldehydes and ketones, amines, and carboxylic acids and their derivatives can be attracted to dissimilar functional groups forming intermolecular bonds. And once again this bonding will potentially effect biologic activity, pharmacokinetic properties, and physical-chemical properties.

EMPIRIC METHOD FOR PREDICTING WATER SOLUBILITY

The presentation above would suggest that functional groups are capable of exhibiting intra- and intermolecular hydrogen bonding in a polyfunctional molecule, which decreases the potential for promoting water solubility. How much weight should be given to each such interaction for individual functional groups? This is a difficult question to answer, but as a general rule, if one is conservative in the amount of solubilizing potential that is given to each functional group, one will find that fairly accurate predictions can be made for polyfunctional molecules.

Now let's look at several examples of how we might use our knowledge of individual functional groups and their bonding and solubilizing potential to predict water solubility of complex molecules. Beginning with the example cited above of α-amino acids such as tyrosine (Fig. 18.3). This molecule has three functional groups: a phenol, an amine, and a carboxylic acid. By a simple summation of the water-solubilizing potential of each functional group, one would predict that the phenol would solubilize 6 to 7 carbon atoms, the amine 6 to 7 carbon atoms, and the carboxyl 5 to 6 carbon atoms, giving a total solubilizing potential of 17 to 20 carbon atoms. Tyrosine contains nine carbons, yet the molecule is soluble to the extent of 0.5%. The explanation for this lack of water solubility can be understood if one

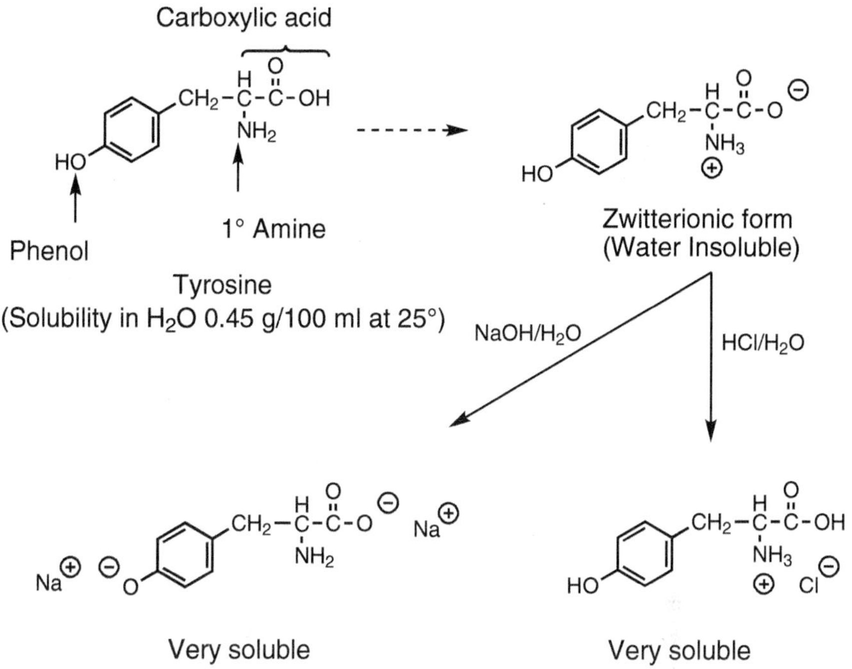

FIGURE 18-3. Solubility of tyrosine in water, aqueous base, and aqueous acid.

recognizes the possibility of intramolecular bonding of the zwitterion (Fig. 18.3). The charged molecule exhibits intramolecular ion-ion bonding, which destroys the ability of these two functional groups to bond to water and the phenol is not capable by itself of dissolving the molecule. This intramolecular bonding can be destroyed by either adding sodium hydroxide or hydrochloric acid to the amino acid, resulting in compounds that are quite water-soluble.

In Table 18.1, the various functional groups that have been discussed are listed with the solubilizing potential of each group when present in a monofunctional molecule and in a polyfunctional molecule. This latter value will be the more useful, since most of the drug molecules to be discussed will be polyfunctional.

The next examples are shown in Figure 18.4. One should recognize the presence of two tertiary amines. If the more liberal solubilizing potential for an amine is used, it might be expected that each amine would have the capability of solubilizing up to 7 carbon atoms, leading to a total potential of dissolving 14 carbon atoms in the molecule. Since the molecule contains 13 carbon atoms, one would predict that the molecule to be soluble. Using the more conservative estimate and allowing three carbons worth of solubility to each amine, a prediction of insoluble would result. It turns out that the molecule is water-soluble. The use of the more liberal estimate in order to obtain the correct results is acceptable in this case because the molecule contains only amines that act alike, not creating any new intermolecular bonds. Also important for this molecule is the fact that both amines

Table 18.1. WATER-SOLUBILIZING POTENTIAL OF ORGANIC FUNCTIONAL GROUPS WHEN PRESENT IN A MONO- OR POLYFUNCTIONAL MOLECULE*

FUNCTIONAL GROUP	MONOFUNCTIONAL MOLECULE	POLYFUNCTIONAL MOLECULE
Alcohol	5 to 6 carbons	3 to 4 carbons
Phenol	6 to 7 carbons	3 to 4 carbons
Ether	4 to 5 carbons	2 carbons
Aldehyde	4 to 5 carbons	2 carbons
Ketone	5 to 6 carbons	2 carbons
Amine	6 to 7 carbons	3 carbons
Carboxylic acid	5 to 6 carbons	3 carbons
Ester	6 carbons	3 carbons
Amide	6 carbons	2 to 3 carbons
Urea, Carbonate, Carbamate		2 carbons

*Water solubility is defined as >1% solubility.

are tertiary amines and tertiary amines are weak dipoles showing little potential for dipole-dipole bonding. Because of the location of the amines intramolecular bonding does not occur.

With paradimethylaminobenzaldehyde (Fig. 18.4), a nine-carbon molecule, the liberal estimate would predict solubility, since the amine is capable of solubilizing up to 7 carbon atoms and an aldehyde could solubilize up to 5 carbon atoms. On the other hand, the conservative estimate would predict insolubility with the

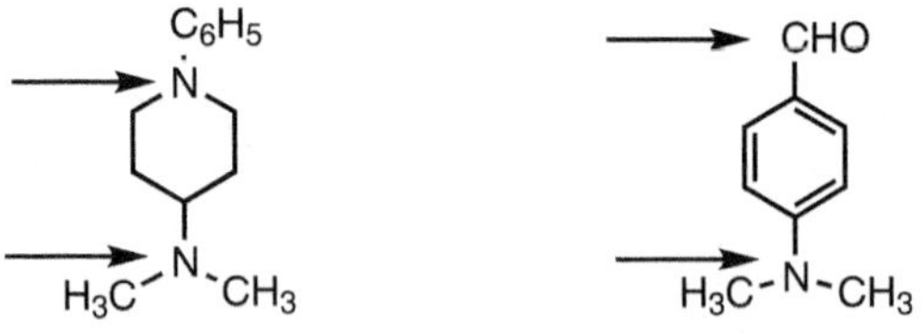

C_6H_5

$C_{13}H_{20}N_2$

$7 + 7 = 14$

$3 + 3 = 6$

Water-soluble

CHO

$C_9H_{11}NO$

$7 + 5 = 12$

$3 + 2 = 5$

Slightly water-soluble

FIGURE 18-4. Prediction of water solubility of organic molecules using mono- and polyfunctional estimates for the functional groups.

amine worth 3 and the aldehyde worth 2 carbon atoms. This molecule is listed as slightly soluble, a result that falls between the two estimates. This simply shows that these are only predictions and, with borderline compounds, may lead to inaccurate results.

The next examples shown in Figure 18.5 lead to a more accurate prediction. In the first compound, one should recognize the presence of three ethers, a phenol, and a tertiary amine. Using the monofunctional solubilizing potential, one would expect enough solubility from these groups to dissolve this 19-carbon compound, since each ether would be assigned 5 carbons, the phenol 7 carbons of solubilizing potential, and the amine 7 carbons worth of solubilizing potential. If one uses the more conservative estimate, which takes into consideration the intra- and intermolecular bonding, each ether contributes 2 carbons with of solubility, while the phenol and amine contribute 3 and 4 carbons worth of solubilizing potential, respectively. The prediction now is that the molecule is insoluble in water, and this turns out to be the case.

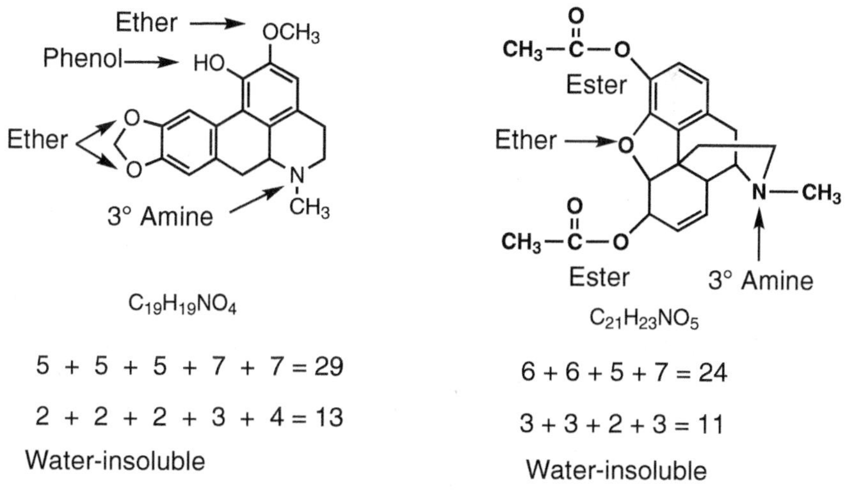

FIGURE 18-5. Prediction of water solubility of organic molecules using mono- and polyfunctional estimates for the functional groups.

The second structure in Figure 18.5 has two esters, an ether, and a 3° amine. Once the functional groups are identified one needs only to assign the solubilizing potential to each group. Again, the monofunctional potentials are inappropriate since this is a polyfunctional molecule and if used would have resulted in a prediction of water solubility. Using the polyfunctional solubilizing potential gives the more accurate prediction of the molecule being water-insoluble. The polyfunctional potential is more appropriate since this molecule would be expected to have both intramolecular and intermolecular bonding.

Additional examples of the empirical approach to predicting water solubility can be found within the problem sets of the Student Workbook CD-ROM.

ANALYTIC METHOD FOR CALCULATING WATER SOLUBILITY

Throughout this presentation, emphasis has been placed on the water-solubilizing properties of the common organic functional groups. This is restated in Table 18.1 with carbon-solubilizing potentials for each functional group, and the use of these values was demonstrated by the examples shown in Figures 18.4 and 18.5. While this approach is empiric, others have attempted to derive an analytic method for calculation of water solubility. One such mathematical approach is based upon the partitioning of a drug between octanol (a standard for lipophilic media) and water. The base-ten logarithm of the partition coefficients is defined as log P. While the measured log P values are a measure of the solubility characteristics of the whole molecule, one can use fragments of the whole molecule and assign a specific hydrophilic-lipophilic value (defined as π value) to each of these fragments. Thus, a calculated log P can be obtained by the sum of the hydrophilic-lipophilic fragments:

$$\log P = \frac{\text{Conc. of Drug in Octanol}}{\text{Conc. of Drug in Water}} \qquad \text{(Eq. 1)}$$

$$\log P_{calc} = \Sigma \pi_{(fragments)} \qquad \text{(Eq. 2)}$$

To use this procedure, the student must fragment the molecule into basic units and assign an appropriate π value corresponding to the atoms or groups of atoms present. Table 18.2 lists the common fragments found in organic molecules and their

Table 18.2. HYDROPHILIC-LIPOPHILIC VALUES (π VALUES) FOR ORGANIC FRAGMENTS

FRAGMENTS	π VALUES
C (aliphatic)	+0.5
C (alkene)	+0.33
Phenyl	+2.0
Cl (halogen)	+0.5
S	+0.0
N (amine)	−1.0
O (hydroxyl, phenol, ether)	−1.0
O_2NO	+0.2
O_2N (aliphatic)	−0.85
O_2N (aromatic)	−0.28
O=C-O	−0.7
O=C-N (other than amine)	−0.7
IMHB	+0.65

π values. Positive values for π mean that the fragment, relative to hydrogen, is lipophilic or favors solubility in octanol. A negative value indicates a hydrophilic group and thus an affinity for water. While the environment of the substituent can influence the π value, such changes are small, and for our purposes this factor can be neglected.

Through the examination of a large number of experimentally obtained log P and solubility values, an arbitrary standard has been adopted whereby those chemicals with a positive log P value over +0.5 are considered water-insoluble (i.e., solubility is less than 3.3% in water—a definition for solubility used by the USP). Log P values less than +0.5 are considered water-soluble.

This method of calculating water solubility has proved quite effective with a large number of organic molecules containing C, Cl, N, and O, but several additional factors may have to be considered for specific drugs. A complicating factor is the influence of intramolecular hydrogen bonding (IMHB) on π values. As discussed in the previous empiric approach to predicting water solubility, IMHB would be expected to decrease water solubility, and, therefore, where IMHB exists, a π value of +0.65 is added to the calculations. An example of using this factor is shown for salicylic acid (Fig. 18.6).

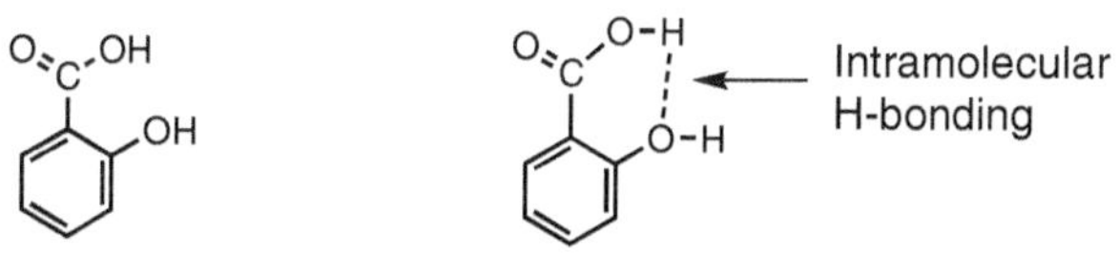

Solubility 0.2%

Calc. log P without IMHB		Calc. log P with IMHB	
Phenyl	+2.0	Phenyl	+2.0
O-H	−1.0	O-H	−1.0
O=C-O	−0.7	O=C-O	−0.7
		IMHB	+0.65
Total	+0.3	Total	+0.95
Prediction	Soluble	Prediction	Insoluble

FIGURE 18-6. Calculation of water solubility of salicylic acid without and with the intramolecular hydrogen bonding (IMHB) factor.

The log P values of a drug with acid or base character are influenced by the pH of the media in which the drug is placed. This is not surprising, since acid or base groups will become ionic under appropriate conditions. Although the π values given in Table 18.2 were obtained under conditions in which the amine, phenol, or carboxylic acid are unionized, which would allow an accurate prediction of log P, observed log Ps at various pH values may not be accurate for water prediction. The experimental log Ps found for procaine are −0.32 (pH 7) and 0.14 (pH 8), both of

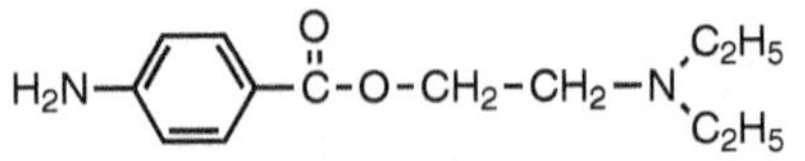

Procaine

Phenyl....................	+2.0
6 - C @ +0.5...........	+3.0
2 - N @ –1.0	–2.0
O=C-O	–0.7
Total.......................	+2.3
Prediction	Insoluble

FIGURE 18-7. Calculation of water solubility of procaine.

which would lead to the prediction that procaine is water-soluble. In fact, procaine is soluble to the extent of 0.5% at pH 7. The calculated log P = +2.3 (Fig. 18.7) correctly predicts that procaine is water insoluble.

Case Study 18.1

You are working the "graveyard" shift in the county hospital pharmacy when a call comes in from the ER. LN, a 21-year-old anorexic woman seriously injured in a car accident, has just been brought in by ambulance. LN is 5'8" and weighs 102 pounds. She is in significant pain, and the physician wants your opinion on which of three opioid analgesics drawn below would be best to use in this situation. The opioid, in salt form, will be administered intravenously.

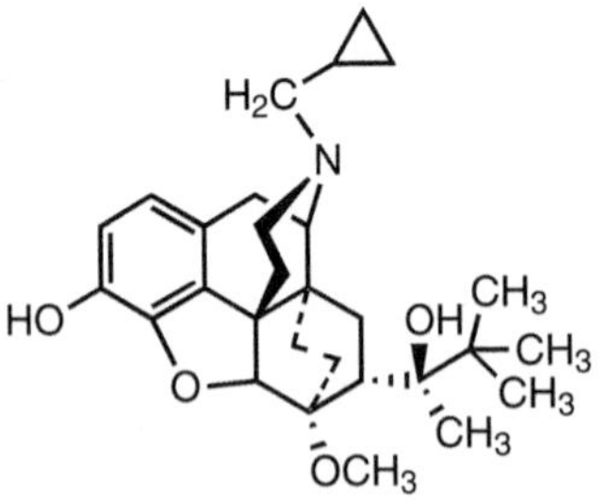

Buprenorphine 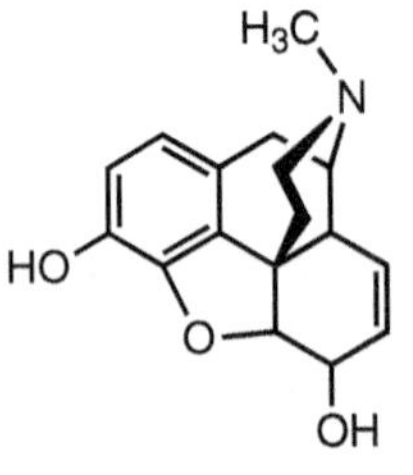   Morphine 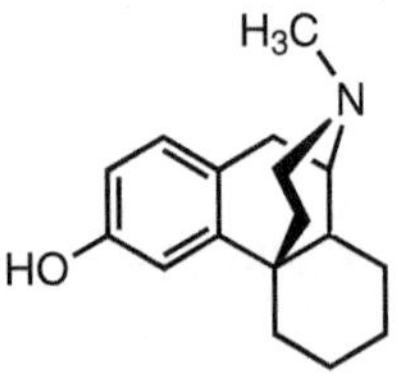   Levorphanol

You inform this physician that opioids are relatively lipophilic structures, and they attempt to get out of the aqueous circulation by distributing into body fat

Case Study 18.1 (continued)

(a peripheral storage site) and brain (the site of action). Drug manufacturers take this into account when establishing the dose. In a person of normal body weight, the amount of drug reaching the brain is enough to induce analgesia, but not enough to cause life-threatening side effects like respiratory depression. The more lipophilic the drug, the more readily it is sequestered into the fat, and the more willingly it will cross the blood-brain barrier from the bloodstream.

After reminding LN's attending of this important pharmacokinetic reality, you evaluate the impact of the functional groups of the three opioid structures on relative water/lipid solubility and make your decision. Which opioid will you recommend for LN?

Case Study 18.2

You are doing an early experiential rotation shadowing in a compounding pharmacy. You are learning that emulsions can be of two main types, that is, oil-in-water (O/W) and water-in oil (W/O). You also learned that O/W emulsions are carriers for lipophilic drugs and W/O emulsions are carriers for hydrophilic drugs. Since the precepting pharmacist knows you like chemistry and have had the course in organic functional groups, he presents you with the following three drugs and asks you if you would emulsify them in O/W or W/O emulsions. By looking at their structures and using the water-solubilizing potential of organic functional groups found in Table 18.1, predict which media you will use for your emulsions.

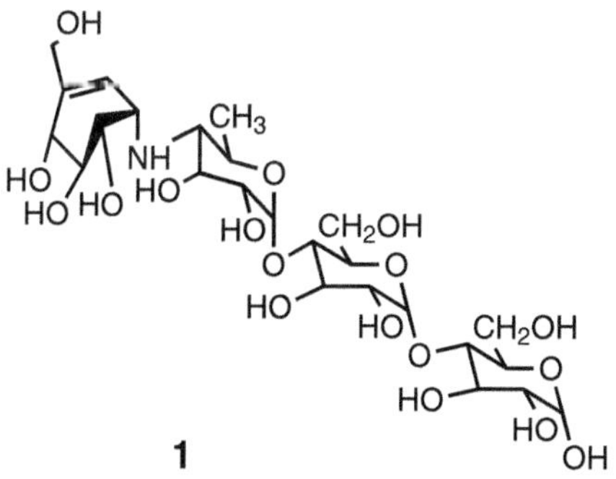

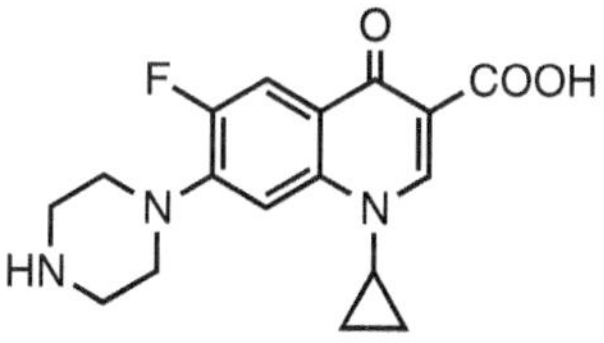

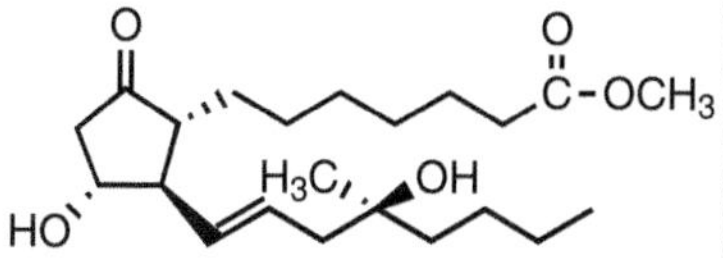

Stereoisomerism — Asymmetric Molecules

A carbon atom substituted with four different substituents does not possess a plane or point of symmetry and as a result is an asymmetric molecule. A carbon atom substituted with two or more of the same substituents has either a plane or point of symmetry and as a result is a symmetric molecule. With the compound 2-methyl-2-butanol, carbon atoms 2, 3, and 4 and the OH and one hydrogen lie in a single plane with the remaining four methyls and two hydrogens symmetrically located above and behind the plane of the page (Fig. A-1). This compound is said to have a plane of symmetry and is a symmetric molecule. On the other hand, 2-butanol does not have a plane of symmetry, is said to be asymmetric, and consists of two nonsuperimposable molecules or a pair of enantiomers. The second enantiomer can be easily generated by reflecting the initial molecule in a mirror as shown in

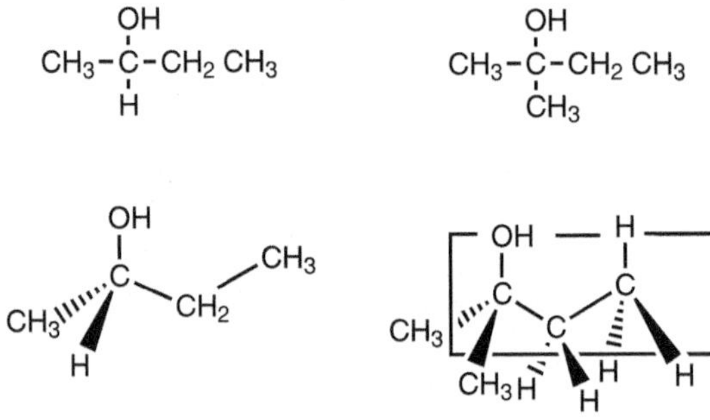

FIGURE A-1. Structure of the asymmetric 2-butanol and the symmetric 2-methyl-2-butanol.

Figure A-2. If the mirror image is rotated by 180°, one can see that the enantiomers are not superimposable. 2-Butanol is said to be a chiral molecule with two enantiomeric forms. What is the significance of chirality? The two enantiomers have the same empirical formula, and behave similarly with the exception that the individual enantiomers will rotate plane polarized light in opposite directions. One of the isomers, when placed in a polarimeter, rotates the plane of polarization to the right (clockwise), is said to be dextrorotatory and is labeled the D isomer or (+) isomer. The other isomer causes a counterclockwise rotation of the plane of polarization

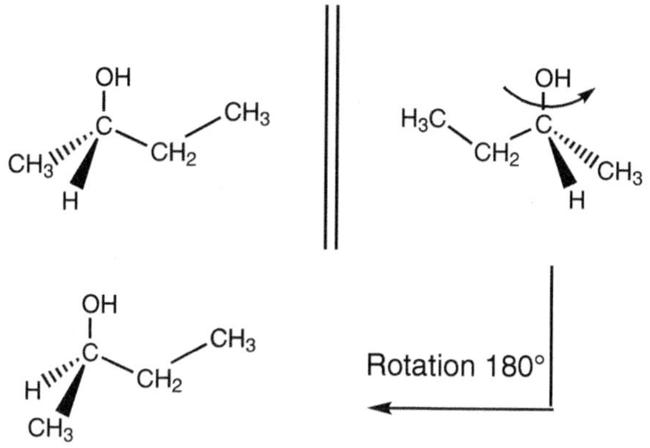

FIGURE A-2. Enantiomers of 2-butanol.

and is thus the levorotatory isomer abbreviated as the L isomer or (−) isomer. The degree of rotation is the same for both enantiomers but in opposite directions. The fact that enantiomers can bend plane polarized light has caused such compounds to be referred to as optically active isomers. If a compound exists as an equal mixture of both isomers, the material is said to be racemic, with a net rotation of polarization of zero. The significance of chirality and its role in medicinal chemistry relates to the fact that chiral molecules are capable of recognizing the difference between two enantiomeric molecules. An example of this relates to the interaction or bonding of a small molecular weight molecule (a drug) with a protein. Enzymes and drug receptor sites are generally proteins that in turn are made up of chiral amino acids. Many chiral enzymes and drug receptors react selectively with one of the enantiomers of a chiral drug, producing a biologic response. The second enantiomer may have little or no biologic activity. One must recognize the presence of a chiral center in a drug molecule and appreciate the importance of this property as it affects biologic activity.

Another aspect of a chiral center should be reviewed and that is their nomenclature. The direction of rotation of plane polarized light is a relative property and does not indicate the absolute configuration around the chiral center. The Cahn–Ingold–Prelog "R" and "S" nomenclature is used to indicate absolute configuration. A set of arbitrary sequence rules assigns to the atoms around the chiral center priorities of 1 through 4, with number 1 being the highest priority. The molecule is then physically rotated so that the number 4 group is placed behind the remaining three groups and farthest from the eye of the viewer. One then notes the direction in which the eye travels in going from groups 1 to 2 to 3. If the direction is clockwise, the molecule is assigned the absolute configuration of R, while if the direction is counterclockwise the center is assigned the S absolute configuration (Fig. A-3). While many sequence rules are used for the many different functional groups encountered in organic chemistry, the one that suffices

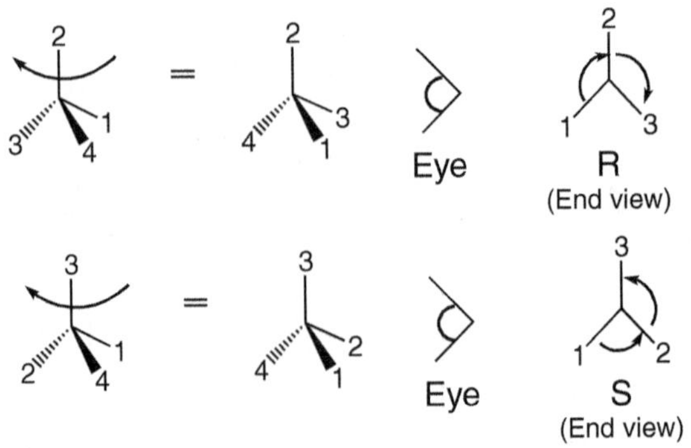

FIGURE A-3. Cahn–Ingold–Prelog method of assigning absolute configuration.

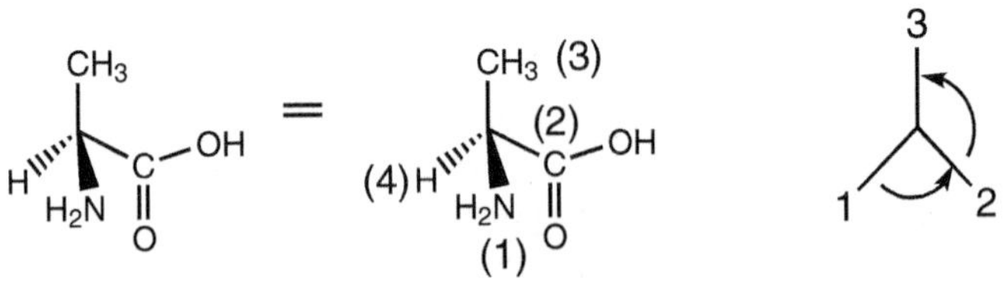

$$N > C\text{-}O > C\text{-}H > H$$

FIGURE A-4. (S)-2-aminopropionic acid [(S)-alanine].

for most situations is that the atom with a higher atomic number precedes a lower atomic number atom. Thus, for the amino acid alanine shown in Figure A-4, the N (atomic No. 7) has higher priority than C (atomic No. 6), which has higher priority than H (atomic No. 1). To differentiate between the CH_3 and the COOH group, one must go to the atoms attached to the carbons, and the O (atomic No. 8) has priority over H.

Acidity and Basicity

B

Throughout the book, considerable emphasis has been placed on the physical-chemical properties of the various functional groups. One of the major physical-chemical properties emphasized has been that of acidity/basicity. If a functional group is acidic, conversion of that group to a salt that can dissociate in water dramatically improves water solubility through ion-dipole bonding. In a similar fashion, if a functional group is basic, it can be converted to a salt by treatment with an acid. If the salt dissociates in water, water solubility will be increased through ion-dipole bonding. Since water solubility is quite important for drug delivery, it is felt that a short review of the concept of acidity and basicity is called for. In addition, a compilation of the important acids and bases, drawn from this book, will be presented in this appendix.

DEFINITIONS OF ACIDS AND BASES

Although there are several definitions for acids and bases, the most useful for our purposes is the Brønsted-Lowry definition. According to this definition, an acid is defined as any substance that can donate a proton; a base is a substance that can accept a proton. Shown here is the reaction of HX with water. HX is donating a proton to water, and HX is therefore an acid. By virtue of the fact that water is accepting the proton, water is a base. The anion, X^-, formed from the acid, HX, is also capable of accepting a proton and is thus defined as the conjugate base of HX. In a similar manner, the hydronium ion, H_3O^+, is a conjugate acid of the base water. In this reaction, there are two conjugate acid-base pairs: the conjugate acid-base pair made up of HX and X^- and the conjugate acid-base pair made up of H_2O and H_3O^+. The Brønsted-Lowry definition of acids and bases necessitates the concept of conjugate acid-base pairs. Indeed, an acid (or base) cannot demonstrate its acidic (or basic) properties unless a base (or acid) is present. In the example shown, HX cannot

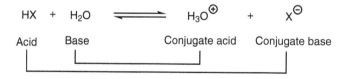

donate its proton unless there is another substance (a base) to accept that proton. Several additional examples of acids and bases are shown in Figure B-1.

Several interesting phenomena should be noted in these examples. Water is acting as a base in the first three examples and as an acid in the latter three examples.

Since water can act as either an acid or a base, it is said to be amphoteric. Also seen in Figure B-1 are examples of compounds that demonstrate another useful definition of a base. Lewis defined a base as an electron-pair donor. This definition is useful in identifying organic bases such as amines. Alkyl and aryl amines are basic by virtue of their ability to donate a pair of electrons.

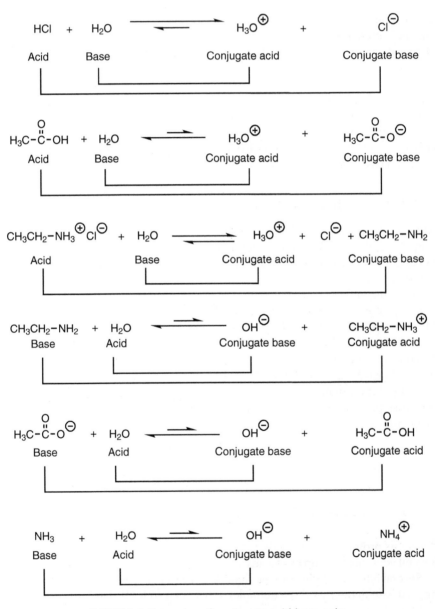

FIGURE B-1. Examples of conjugate acid-base pairs.

RELATIVE STRENGTHS OF ACIDS AND BASES

The strength of an acid depends on its ability to donate a proton. The strong acids have a strong tendency to give up a proton, while the weak acids have little tendency to give up a proton. Virtually all organic compounds could be considered acids. A compound like methane (CH_4) can give up a proton when treated with a sufficiently strong base. However, when dealing with water as the pharmaceutical solvent and with the intention of creating water-soluble salts, the list of acids is greatly reduced. Thus, the alcohol functional group, which an organic chemist may consider an acid, from our standpoint is considered a neutral functional group. The same limitations must be placed on the base. Many compounds that a chemist would consider basic will not give stable salts when placed in water. Therefore, the drug list of basic functional groups is quite limited.

$$\text{Strong acid:} \quad HX \ + \ H_2O \ \rightleftharpoons \ H_3O^{\oplus} \ + \ X^{\ominus}$$

$$\text{Weak acid:} \quad HX \ + \ H_2O \ \rightleftharpoons \ H_3O^{\oplus} \ + \ X^{\ominus}$$

The discussion of the relative strength of an acid really becomes a discussion of the nature of the dissociation equilibrium for the acid in water. A strong acid is one that has a strong tendency to dissociate. The strong acids commonly used in pharmacy are nearly completely dissociated in water (e.g., H_2SO_4, HCl, HNO_3). If a compound is a strong acid, then its conjugate base is weak. The weak acids are

$$HCl \ + \ H_2O \ \longrightarrow \ H_3O^{\oplus} \ + \ Cl^{\ominus}$$

| Strong acid | Base | | Weak conjugate acid | Weak conjugate base |

those compounds that have a poor tendency to dissociate in water (e.g., carboxylic acids, phenols, sulfonamides, imides). Such compounds are characterized as having relatively strong conjugate bases. In all cases, the equilibrium will tend to favor the direction that gives the weaker acid and the weaker base.

$$H_3C\text{-}\overset{O}{\overset{\|}{C}}\text{-}OH \ + \ H_2O \ \longrightarrow \ H_3O^{\oplus} \ + \ H_3C\text{-}\overset{O}{\overset{\|}{C}}\text{-}O^{\ominus}$$

| Weak acid | Weak base | | Strong conjugate acid | Strong conjugate base |

In a similar fashion, the relative strength of a base depends upon the ability of the chemical to give up a hydroxyl or the tendency to accept a proton. Table B-1 is a listing of common acids and bases in order of acidity. The table actually becomes compressed when water is specified as our solvent. All of the acids above the hydronium ion show a reduction in apparent acidity because of the leveling effect in water. Since the strong acids (e.g., H_2SO_4, HCl, HNO_3) are nearly completely

Table B-1. ACID-BASE CHART

ACIDS

H_2SO_4

HCl

HNO_3

$H_3O^{\oplus}$

RCO_2H

ArOH

RSO_2NH_2

$-\overset{O}{\overset{\|}{C}}-\overset{H}{\overset{|}{N}}-\overset{O}{\overset{\|}{C}}-$

H_2O

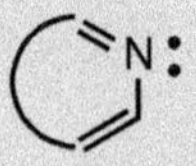

ArNH$_2$

$R-\overset{NH}{\overset{\|}{C}}-NH_2$

Alkyl$-NH_2$

$R\,HN-\overset{NH}{\overset{\|}{C}}-NH_2$

NaOH, KOH

BASES

Increasing Basicity ←

Increasing Acidity →

dissociated in water to form hydronium ions, their acidities become equal in water and the hydronium ion becomes the strongest ion. The leveling effect also affects strong bases. In water, the strongest base that can exist is the hydroxide ion; therefore, sodium hydroxide and potassium hydroxide, which completely dissociate, become equivalent in basicity.

A brief reminder about the acid-base properties of water, which can dissociate to form hydronium ion and hydroxide ion, is shown. The hydronium ions and hydroxide ions formed by this dissociation are present in equal concentrations (i.e., there is no excess of either hydronium ions or hydroxide ions). Hence, water is neutral.

$$H_2O \; + \; H_2O \; \rightleftharpoons \; H_3O^{\oplus} \; + \; OH^{\ominus}$$

Acid   Base   Conjugate acid   Conjugate base

REACTION OF AN ACID WITH A BASE IN WATER

The reaction of an acid with a base in water is known as a neutralization reaction. When a strong acid reacts with a strong base, one actually finds that the reaction consists of hydronium ions formed by the acid reacting with the hydroxide ions formed by the base. The neutralization reaction between a strong acid and a strong base results in an aqueous solution that is neutral. The anion of an acid and the cation of a base do not react with each other but are simply present as a salt. The situation is not the same when a weak acid is neutralized by a strong base. In the

$$HNO_3 \; + \; H_2O \; \rightleftharpoons \; H_3O^{\oplus} \; + \; NO_3^{\ominus}$$

$$KOH \; + \; H_2O \; \rightleftharpoons \; K^{\oplus} \; + \; OH^{\ominus}$$

$$H_3O^{\oplus} + OH^{\ominus} + K^{\oplus} + NO_3^{\ominus} \longrightarrow 2\,H_2O + K^{\oplus} + NO_3^{\ominus}$$

acid-base reaction between acetic acid and sodium hydroxide, sodium acetate, the weak conjugate base of acetic acid, and water, the weak conjugate acid of the hydroxide ion, are formed. The sodium acetate will partially dissociate in water, however, to afford acetic acid and hydroxide ion. This will result in a slight excess of hydroxide ion in solution when the "neutralization" reaction is complete, and the pH of the solution will be greater than 7, or alkaline.

$$CH_3COOH \; + \; NaOH \; \rightleftharpoons \; H_2O \; + \; CH_3COO^{\ominus}Na^{\oplus}$$

Weak acid   Strong base   Weak acid   Weak base

$$CH_3COO^{\ominus}Na^{\oplus} + H_2O \; \rightleftharpoons \; CH_3COOH \; + \; OH^{\ominus} + Na^{\oplus}$$

Base   Acid   Conjugate acid   Conjugate base

An analogous situation occurs in neutralization reactions between weak bases and strong acids, except that the final solution is acidic. In this example, the dissociation of the salt formed during the neutralization reaction produces hydronium ion. The resulting solution from this neutralization reaction will have a pH less than 7 (acidic), in that the strength of the hydronium ion is more acidic than the amine is basic. The amount of hydronium ion formed depends on the extent of dissociation of the amine salt.

$$(CH_3CH_2)_3N \ + \ HCl \longrightarrow (CH_3CH_2)_3NH^{\oplus} \ + \ Cl^{\ominus}$$

Weak base   Strong acid   Weak acid   Weak base

$$(CH_3CH_2)_3NH^{\oplus} + \ H_2O \rightleftharpoons (CH_3CH_2)_3N \ + \ H_3O^{\oplus}$$

Acid   Base   Conjugate base   Conjugate acid

This concept is quite important if one considers what happens to the pH of water if a sodium or potassium salt of an organic acid is dissolved in water. The organic anion is the conjugate base of a weak acid, and when placed in water the pH of the solution becomes alkaline. Another way of considering this is that, in water, one has the salt of a weak acid and a strong base. Since the strong base is farther up the pH scale than the weak acid is down the scale, the net sum of this is that the pH remains greater than 7 (Fig. B-2). When a sulfate, chloride, or nitrate salt of an organic base

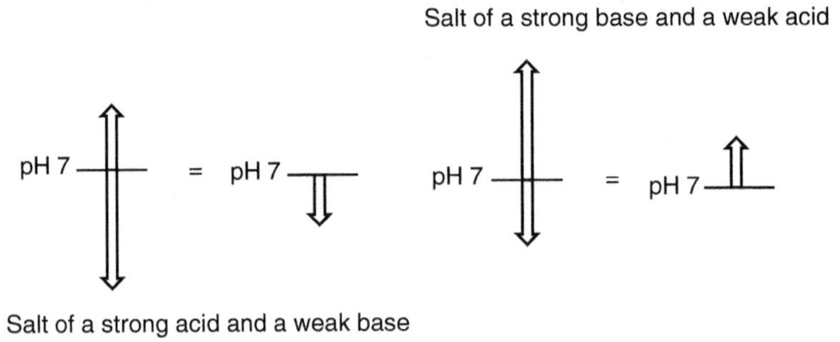

Salt of a strong base and a weak acid

Salt of a strong acid and a weak base

FIGURE B-2. Diagrammatic representation for predicting pH of an aqueous media after addition of a water-soluble salt to water.

is dissolved in water, one has a salt of a weak base and a strong acid. The strong acid is farther down the pH scale than the base is up the scale, and the pH of the solution therefore is below 7. Using this concept, one can successfully predict the pH of many salts after dissolving the salt in water (Table B-2). The clue to predicting the correct answer is in being able to recognize whether one is dealing with salts of strong acids and weak bases or weak acids and strong bases. A rule of thumb that is most helpful is that the strong acids are hydrochloric, sulfuric, nitric, perchloric, and phosphoric acid. All other acids are weak. The strong bases are sodium hydroxide and potassium hydroxide. All other bases are weak.

Table B-2. DISSOCIATION IN WATER

				PREDICTION
$ZnCl_2$ +	$2 H_2O \rightleftharpoons$	$H_3O^{\oplus}$ + $Cl^{\ominus}$	+ $Zn(OH)Cl$	Acidic
Lewis acid	Base	Strong acid	Weak base	
Na_2CO_3 +	$2 H_2O \rightleftharpoons$	$2 Na^{\oplus}$ + $2 OH^{\ominus}$	+ H_2CO_3	Basic
Base	Acid	Strong base	Weak acid	
$Ca(NO_3)_2$ +	$2 H_2O \rightleftharpoons$	$H_3O^{\oplus}$ + $NO_3^{\ominus}$	+ $Ca(OH)NO_3$	Acidic
Base	Acid	Strong acid	Weak base	

$$\text{(imide)}N^{\ominus}\ Na^{\oplus} + H_2O \rightleftharpoons Na^{\oplus} + OH^{\ominus} + \text{(imide)}N-H \qquad \text{Basic}$$

Base	Acid	Strong base	Weak acid	

ACIDIC AND BASIC ORGANIC FUNCTION GROUPS

This section presents, in a single location, a synopsis of most of the organic acids and bases that are important in drugs as potential salt-forming sites. As stated earlier, nearly all organic compounds could be considered potentially acidic, but put in the context of water as the solvent, only a few functional groups are acidic enough to be of practical value.

Table B-3 lists the organic acids that have been reviewed in this book. Although sulfonic acids are the most acidic of the "organic" functional groups, few drugs contain them. The carboxylic acids are the most acidic organic functional groups found in drug molecules. The nature of the "R" group strongly influences the strength of this acidity (for a review of this influence, see Chap. 11).

When "R" is an electron-withdrawing group, relative to hydrogen, the acidity increases, and when "R" is an electron-releasing group, relative to hydrogen, the acidity decreases. The effects of "R" on acidity, inductively or by resonance, stabilize or destabilize the carboxylate anion, respectively. The sulfonamide is an acidic functional group provided that the sulfonamide is unsubstituted or monosubstituted. A disubstituted sulfonamide does not have a proton on the nitrogen and cannot be acidic. Phenols are relatively weak acids that can be strongly influenced by the nature of the aromatic substituent (see Chap. 7). Electron-withdrawing groups in the para or meta position increase acidity by resonance or a combination of resonance and inductive action. Electron-releasing groups likewise reduce acidity

Table B-3. ORDER OF ACIDITY OF ORGANIC ACIDS

ACIDS	ACIDITY (pKa)
$R-SO_3H$	1
$R-COOH$	4–5
$Ar-SO_2NHR$	6–9
$Ar-OH$	8–11
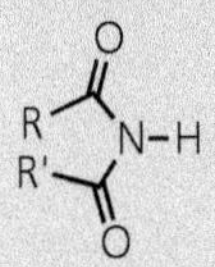 (imide structure)	8–10

because such groups destabilize the phenolate anion. Finally, common to a number of heterocycles is the imide functional group, which must have a proton on the nitrogen to be acidic.

All of the organic acids (with the exception of sulfonic acid) are weak acids, which is to say that, in water, the equilibrium will favor the undissociated molecule. This also explains why salts of organic acids and strong bases, when dissolved in water, produce an appreciable quantity of hydroxide ion, and the aqueous solution is alkaline. The degree of alkalinity will depend on the strength of the acid. Alkaline metal salts of phenols will result in a very basic aqueous solution, while alkaline metal salts of carboxylic acids are less basic.

$$Y-H \; + \; H_2O \; \longrightarrow \; H_3O^{\oplus} \; + \; Y^{\ominus}$$

Weak acid   Weak base   Strong acid   Strong base

Table B-4 lists the organic bases that have been reviewed in this book. Guanidines are the most basic organic functional group, followed by the alkylamines. Within the class of alkylamines the usual order of basicity is secondary amines are more basic than tertiary amines, which are more basic than primary amines. Aromatic amines are significantly (10^{-10}) less basic than alkylamines (10^{-4}), owing to the fact that electron-releasing groups (alkyls) increase basicity, while electron-withdrawing groups (aryls) reduce basicity (see Chap. 10). Aromatic heterocycles containing a nitrogen with a pair of nonbonding electrons are also basic; however, these compounds are weak bases.

$$B\!:\; + \; H_2O \; \longrightarrow \; BH^{\oplus} \; + \; OH^{\ominus}$$

Weak base   Weak acid   Strong acid   Strong base

Table B-4. ORDER OF BASICITY OF ORGANIC BASES

BASES	BASICITY (pKa) (CONJUGATE ACID)
$R-HN-\overset{\overset{\displaystyle NH}{\|\|}}{C}-NH_2$	~13
$R-NH_2$; R_2-NH ; R_3-N	10–11
$R-\overset{\overset{\displaystyle NH}{\|\|}}{C}-NH_2$	9–10
$Ar-NH_2$	1–5
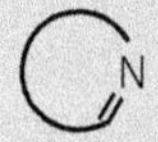 $\bigcirc\!\!\!N$	1–4

(Includes pyridine, imidazole, etc.)

All the organic bases are weak bases, which is to say that in water the equilibrium will favor the free base. Thus, when salts of the organic bases made with strong acids are dissolved in water, an appreciable quantity of hydronium ion will exist and the pH of the aqueous solution will be acidic, the degree of acidity depending on the strength of the base.

Drug Metabolism

INTRODUCTION

The biologic transformation of a drug molecule by enzymes present in the body is commonly referred to as drug metabolism. The process of drug metabolism is usually considered to be a process that leads to detoxification and increased water solubility. In actual fact, metabolism as a chemical transforming process can lead to an increase in toxicity, an activation or deactivation of the biologic action, and in some cases a decrease in water solubility. In addition, drugs represent only one small group of substrates that may undergo metabolism. Any substance foreign to the body can potentially be metabolized after entering the body. A more general term for exogenous substances is the term *xenobiotics*. Xenobiotics represent any foreign chemical and include intentional and unintentional food additives (i.e., herbicides and pesticides), volatile chemicals (i.e., substances in cigarette smoke), chemicals in the drinking water, environmental pollutants in the home and the workplace, as well as drugs. Finally, xenobiotic metabolism, while primarily occurring in the liver, may also occur at extrahepatic sites, including intestine (both within the lumen and the intestinal mucosa), kidney, lungs, nervous tissue, and plasma.

METABOLIC ENZYMES

Xenobiotic metabolism is generally divided into two types of reactions, referred to as phase 1 reactions and phase 2 reactions. Phase 1 reactions include oxidation, reduction, and hydrolysis reactions. These reactions generally involve introduction of a new functional group into the molecule. Phase 2 reactions, which normally follow phase 1, involve conjugation reactions such as acetylation, sulfation, glucuronidation, and conjugation with amino acids. Generally, conjugation reactions lead to inactivation of drug molecules. In many instances xenobiotic metabolism involves a combination of both phase 1 and phase 2 reactions. In any case, xenobiotic metabolism can be predicted and relies on the nature of the functional group or groups present in the organic molecule.

Oxygenase Enzymes

CYTOCHROME P450

A major oxidative enzyme system, and the most studied human enzyme system, is the cytochrome P450 monooxygenase family of enzymes (commonly abbreviated as CYP450). Found in the smooth endoplasmic reticulum of the liver, as well as in some extrahepatic tissue, CYP450 is a very complex enzyme made up of iron-protoporphyrin, NADPH, flavin protein, phospholipids, phosphatidylcholine, and molecular oxygen. CYP450 monooxygenase is not a single enzyme, but instead a family of closely related isoforms. A large number of different isoforms of CYP450 have been identified, each showing a different degree of selectivity and range of activity towards various xenobiotics. It appears that at least eight isoforms of CYP450 play important roles in drug metabolism. Genetic variation appears to play a role in defining the content of each isoform present in human beings and may account for the variations and extent of drug metabolism seen in individual patients. Scientists are just beginning to understand and characterize the structural requirements for selectivity associated with the isoforms of CYP450. The emerging area of pharmacogenomics (i.e., the selection of the right drug for the right patient) can be expected to rely heavily on defining the genetic makeup of CYP450 isoforms of individuals. For a more detailed look at this family of enzymes, their mechanisms of metabolism, and the potential for drug-drug interaction, the reader is referred to *Foye's Principles of Medicinal Chemistry*, 6th ed. Chapter 10.

CYP450 CATALYZED REACTIONS

The common metabolic oxidation reactions involving CYP450 are shown in Table C-1. Oxidation of hydrocarbons is usually dependent upon the nature of the hydrocarbon. While aromatic hydroxylation is quite common, the oxidation of an alkane or alkene is not very common. Oxidation of the alkane carbon adjacent to an aromatic ring is more likely to occur than other sites of alkane oxidation. Alkene metabolism of natural substrates is more likely than is oxidation of alkene xenobiotics.

Dealkylation of short straight chain ethers and amines is a common reaction catalyzed by CYP450. In the case of ethers, it is common for methyl, ethyl, or propyl aryl ethers to be dealkylated, giving rise to phenols and formaldehyde, acetylaldehyde, or propanaldehyde, respectively. Primary amines undergo deamination, while secondary and tertiary short chain amines undergo dealkylation, giving ammonia, a primary amine, or a secondary amine, respectively. Deamination and dealkylation are both identical processes.

Finally, thioethers are oxidized by CYP450 enzymes, leading to a sulfoxide, a single oxidation, or a sulfone, a second oxidation. While thioethers are prone to this type of oxidation, CYP450 is not the usual catalyst for this reaction (see below).

Since the CYP450 family of enzymes are common metabolizing enzymes for a wide variety of xenobiotics, it should not be surprising to find drug-drug, drug-food, and drug-environmental chemical interactions, which will be generically referred to as "drug-drug" interactions. These "drug-drug" interactions may result from more than one xenobiotic interacting with the same CYP450 isoform. One simple explanation for why such interactions can occur is shown for two chemical substances, D_1 and D_2, which react with the same subfamily of CYP450. If $K_1 >> K_2$, then D_1 will be metabolized in preference to D_2, leaving unexpectedly high levels of unmetabolized D_2. A large number of drugs are recognized as inhibitors of specific subfamilies of CYP450. Thus, through this or similar

Table C-1. METABOLIC OXIDATION/REDUCTION REACTIONS

SUBSTRATE	ENZYME	PRODUCT	CHAPTER REFERENCE	OCCURRENCE
Alkane	CYP450	Alcohol	2	Uncommon
Alkene	CYP450	Peroxide	3	Uncommon
Aromatic ring	CYP450	Phenol	4	Common
Alcohol	ADH	Aldehyde/ketone	6	Common
Ether	CYP450	Phenol/ Aldehyde	8	Common
Aldehyde/ketone	ADH	1°/2° alcohol	9	Uncommon
Aldehyde	Aldehyde dehydrogenase	Carboxylic acid	9	Common
1° Amine	CYP450	Aldehyde	10	Common
2°/3° Amine	CYP450	1°/2° amine	10	Common
	FMO	Hydroxylamines		Common
3° Alkylamine	FMO	N-oxide		Common
Ester/amide/ carbonate/carbamate	Hydrolase	Carboxylic acid	12	Common
Thioether	CYP450	Sulfoxide/ Sulfone	14	Uncommon
	FMO	Sulfoxide/ Sulfone	14	Common
Thiol	FMO	Disulfide		Common

mechanisms of enzyme inhibition, a "drug-drug" interaction will occur. Another mechanism of "drug-drug" interaction occurs if a particular substance can induce an increase in activity of a specific CYP450 enzyme. This type of "drug-drug" interaction will lead to an unexpected decrease in the levels of a particular drug, thus reducing the biologic effectiveness of the drug (see *Foye's Principles of Medicinal Chemistry*, 6th ed., Chap. 10).

$$D_1 \xrightarrow[K_1]{CYP450} \overset{OH}{\underset{|}{D_1}}$$

$$D_2 \xrightarrow[K_2]{CYP450} \overset{OH}{\underset{|}{D_2}}$$

FLAVIN MONOOXYGENASE

Flavin monooxygenase (FMO) is a microsomal enzyme with a limited capacity to oxidize xenobiotic substrates. FMO oxidizes alkyl and aryl amines and thiols and thioethers. Tertiary alkylamines are oxidized to N-oxides, while secondary alkylamines, N,N-dialkylarylamines, and N-alkylarylamines form hydroxylamines.

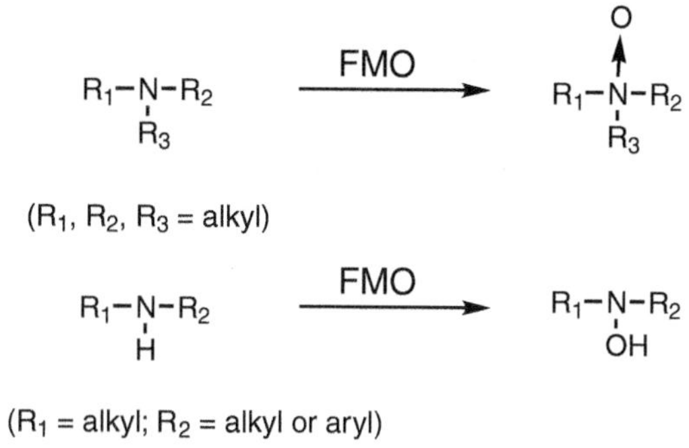

$$R_1-\underset{\underset{R_3}{|}}{N}-R_2 \quad \xrightarrow{\text{FMO}} \quad R_1-\underset{\underset{R_3}{|}}{\overset{\overset{O}{\uparrow}}{N}}-R_2$$

(R_1, R_2, R_3 = alkyl)

$$R_1-\underset{\underset{H}{|}}{N}-R_2 \quad \xrightarrow{\text{FMO}} \quad R_1-\underset{\underset{OH}{|}}{N}-R_2$$

(R_1 = alkyl; R_2 = alkyl or aryl)

The oxidation of sulfur-containing drugs is confined to thiols, which are oxidized to disulfides, and thioethers, which are oxidized to sulfoxides or sulfones. While thioethers can also be oxidized via CYP450, in most cases this type of metabolism occurs through the intervention of FMO.

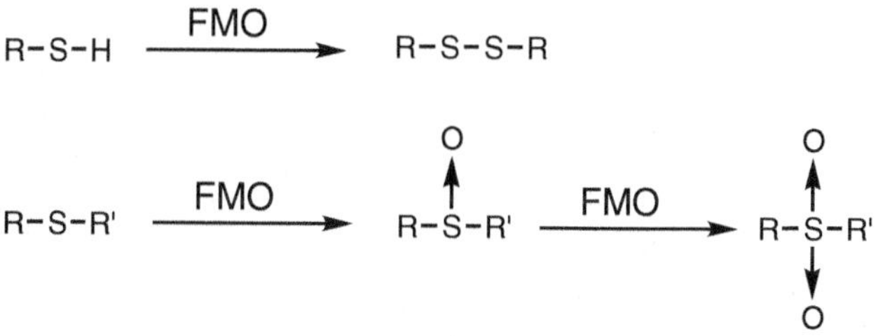

$$R-S-H \quad \xrightarrow{\text{FMO}} \quad R-S-S-R$$

$$R-S-R' \quad \xrightarrow{\text{FMO}} \quad R-\overset{\overset{O}{\uparrow}}{S}-R' \quad \xrightarrow{\text{FMO}} \quad R-\underset{\underset{O}{\downarrow}}{\overset{\overset{O}{\uparrow}}{S}}-R'$$

ALCOHOL DEHYDROGENASE

Alcohol dehydrogenase (ADH), a soluble enzyme found in the cytosol, is a non-hepatic enzyme capable of oxidizing primary and to a lesser extent secondary alcohols to aldehydes and ketones, respectively. While CYP450 is known to also have the ability of oxidizing selected alcohols to aldehydes, alcohol dehydrogenase appears to be the major alcohol-oxidizing enzyme. Alcohol dehydrogenase is also capable of reducing aldehydes and ketones to alcohols, although this does not appear to be as common a reaction.

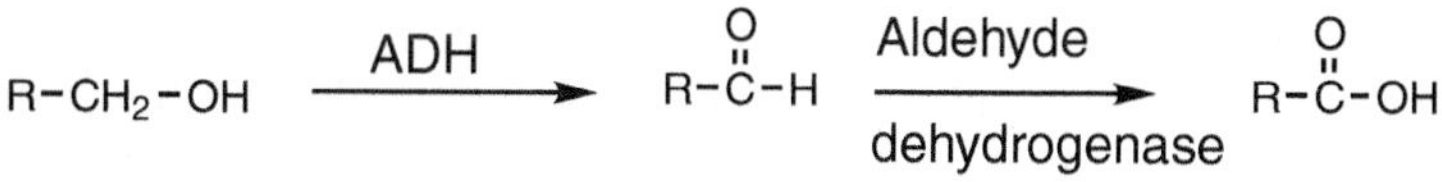

$$R-CH_2-OH \quad \xrightarrow{\text{ADH}} \quad R-\overset{\overset{O}{\|}}{C}-H \quad \xrightarrow[\text{dehydrogenase}]{\text{Aldehyde}} \quad R-\overset{\overset{O}{\|}}{C}-OH$$

ALDEHYDE DEHYDROGENASE

There are a number of enzymes with the ability to catalyze the oxidation of an aldehyde to the corresponding carboxylic acid. Such enzymes are collectively categorized as aldehyde dehydrogenases. Included in this group is the enzyme ADH. These enzymes are commonly found in the cytoplasm.

Hydrolase Enzymes

Another collection of enzymes are those that generically may be called hydrolases. These enzymes attack the functional derivatives of carboxylic acids, leading to hydrolysis. Examples of such enzymes are carboxyesterases, arylesterases, cholinesterase, and serine endopeptidases. These enzymes are found in a wide variety of tissues and fluids. The hydrolase enzymes tend to be more effective in hydrolyzing esters than amides, but amidase enzymes do exist that break down amides to a carboxylic acid and an amine.

Amide hydrolysis tends to occur more commonly with highly lipophilic amides.

Conjugation Reactions

Phase 2 reactions consist of reactions in which new chemical bonds are formed between an organic functional group and a substrate such as glucuronic acid, sulfuric acid, acetic acid, or methyl groups. Generally, one thinks of a conjugation reaction as one that leads to metabolites with increased water solubility, but if one considers acetylation and methylation as conjugation reactions, it can be seen that water solubility may actually decrease. Also, it has been generally thought that conjugation of an organic functional group leads to loss of biologic activity, but recent examples have shown that in some cases the conjugates have increased activity. In most cases the conjugation reactions require the action of a cofactor to complete the reaction. The substrate and an endogenous molecule are brought together, leading to the formation of a new chemical bond. A phase 2 conjugation reaction can follow an initial phase 1 reaction, but it is not uncommon for a phase 2 reaction to occur as the only metabolic reaction. Also, it is possible that multiple conjugation reactions can occur to the same substrate, although this is unlikely since if the water solubility of the initial conjugation metabolite is high the product will be rapidly excreted, thus preventing further metabolism.

GLUCURONIDATION

Glucuronidation consists of the addition of D-glucuronic acid to a variety of substrates, including alcohols, phenols, primary, secondary and occasionally tertiary amines, and carboxylic acids (Table C-2). The glucuronic acid is transferred to the substrate from the cofactor uridine-5′-diphospho-α-D-glucuronic acid (UDPGA). The enzyme responsible for catalyzing this reaction is a UDP-glucuronosyl transferase, which like the CYP450 represents a family of enzymes. These transferases are found in the endoplasmic reticulum of the liver and in

Table C-2. METABOLIC CONJUGATION REACTIONS

CONJUGATION REACTION	SUBSTRATE	CHAPTER REFERENCE	OCCURRENCE
Glucuronidation			
	Alcohol	6	Common
	Phenol	7	Common
	1°/2° Amine	10	Common
	3° Amine	10	Uncommon
	Carboxylic acid	11	Common
Sulfation			
	Alcohol	6	Common
	Phenol	7	Common
	1°/2° Amine	10	Uncommon
Acetylation			
	Arylamine	10	Common
	Phenol	7	Common
Methylation			Common
	Alcohol	6	Common
	Phenol	7	Common
	Thiol		Common

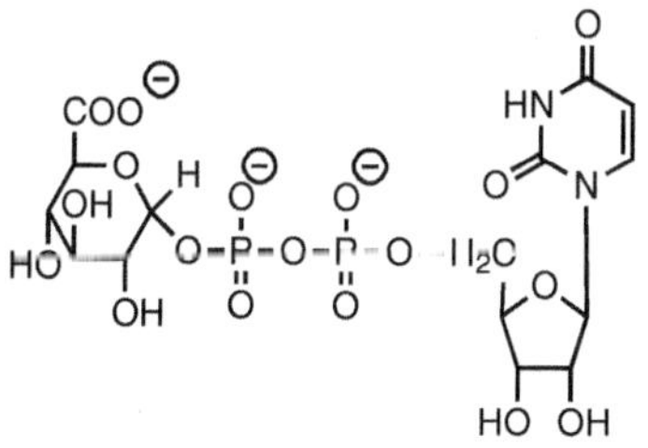

Uridine-5'-diphospho-α-D-glucuronic acid
(UDPGA)

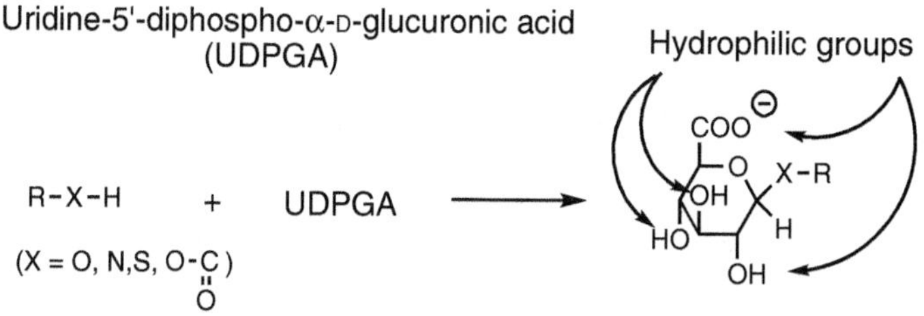

Hydrophilic groups

R–X–H + UDPGA ⟶

(X = O, N,S, O-C)
               ‖
               O

Glucuronide

epithelial cells of the intestine. As would be expected, glucuronidation will greatly improve water solubility of the metabolite through the presence of multiple alcohols and the carboxylic acid group present in the glucuronide. The latter group may be partially ionized at physiologic pH.

SULFATION

Sulfation consists of the addition of sulfuric acid to a variety of substrates, including alcohols, phenol, and to a lesser extent primary and secondary amines (see Table C-2). The sulfuric acid is transferred to the substrate from the cofactor 3'-phosphoadenosine-5'-phosphosulfate (PAPS). The enzymes responsible for catalyzing these reactions are again a family of transferases, the sulfotransferases. These transferases are found primarily in hepatic tissue. Water solubility of the sulfate conjugate is greatly increased since the sulfate is nearly completely ionized at physiologic pH.

3'-Phosphoadenosine-5'-phosphosulfate
(PAPS)

R−X−H   +   PAPS   ⟶

(X = O, N)

Hydrophilic ion-dipole

Sulfate

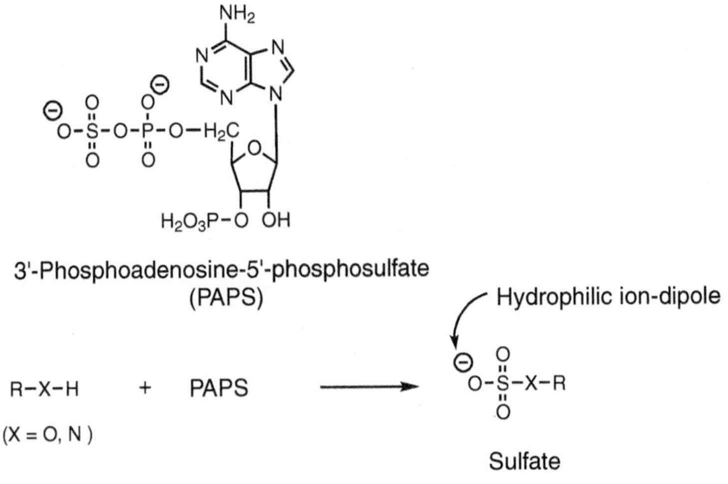

ACETYLATION

Acetylation consists of the addition of an acetate to primary aryl amines (common reaction) and to a lesser extent primary alkyl amines (see Table C-2). The acetate is transferred to the substrate from the cofactor acetylcoenzyme A (acetyl-CoA). The enzymes responsible for catalyzing these reactions are again a family of transferases, the N-acetyltransferases. These transferases are found primarily in hepatic tissue. Depending on the genetic makeup of the patient, the acetylation may be a fast reaction or a slow reaction. Slow acetylators will have higher blood levels of the substrate, while fast acetylators will have higher blood levels of the metabolite. Acetylation products usually show a decrease in water solubility.

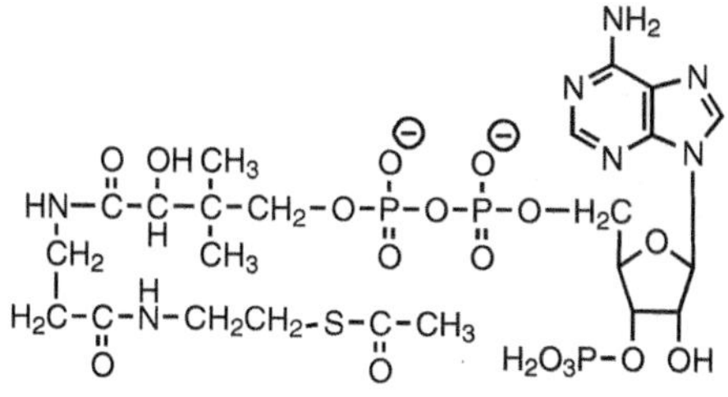

Acetylcoenzyme A (Acetyl-CoA)

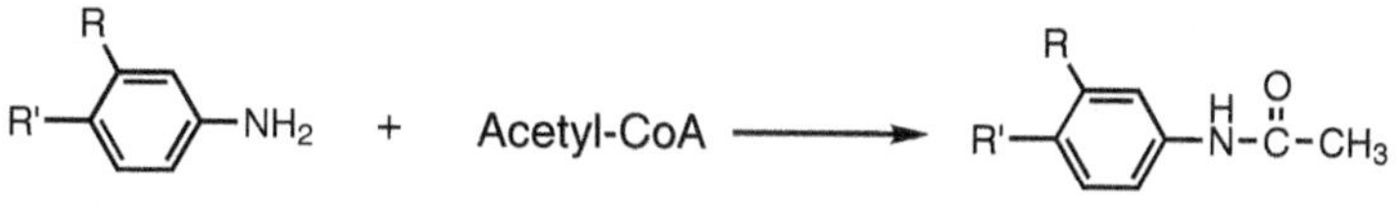

Acetylated metabolite

METHYLATION

Methylation consists of the addition of a methyl group to primarily alcohols, phenols, amines, and thiols (see Table C-2). The methyl is transferred to the substrate from the cofactor S-adenosyl-L-methionine (SAM). The enzymes responsible for catalyzing these reactions are again a family of O-, N-, and S-methyltransferases. Methylation products usually show a decrease in water solubility. Methylation reactions are quite common with endogenous substrates such as norepinephrine and dopamine and drugs that have structural similarities to the natural endogenous metabolites.

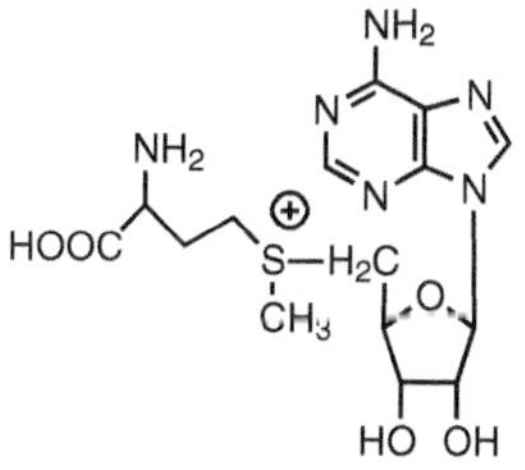

S-Adenosyl-L-methionine
(SAM)

Methylation

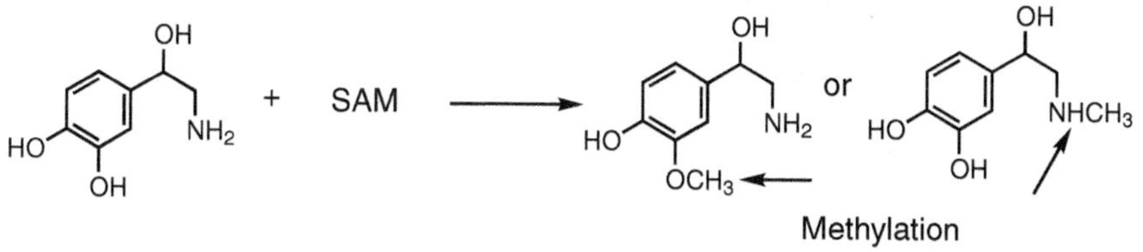

Learning Objectives

NOMENCLATURE

Students should be able to:

1. Identify the organic functional groups present in drug molecules.
2. Correctly identify or draw the general structure of an organic functional group from its generic name.
3. Identify a heterocyclic nucleus given its commonly used nomenclature.
4. Identify and assign stereochemical nomenclature to individual functional groups and to functional groups within polyfunctional molecules.

PHYSICAL-CHEMICAL PROPERTIES AND METABOLISM

Students should be able to:

5. Assign hydrophilic or hydrophobic (lipophilic) properties to every organic functional group.
6. Assign a number representing the degree of water-solubilizing potential to each organic functional group.
7. Define and give the characteristic properties of the various types of chemical bonding that can occur between a functional group and itself, water, and octanol.
8. Rank order the strength of the various types of intermolecular bonding (van der Waal—London, dipole-dipole, ion-dipole, ion-ion bonding) that organic functional group possesses.
9. Define acidity and basicity.
10. Assign pH characteristics to individual organic functional groups (i.e., acidic, basic, neutral).
11. Identify common salts that can form at individual organic functional groups and predict the water-solubilizing properties of the salts.
12. Arrange organic functional groups in order of increasing or decreasing acidity (decreasing basicity or increasing basicity).
13. List chemical instability (or stability) characteristics common to drug formulations for each organic functional group and indicate the likelihood of an in vitro reaction occurring.
14. Draw/identify the products resulting from in vitro chemical instability of an organic functional group.

15. Predict and draw/identify the structure(s) of phase I and/or phase II metabolites formed from individual organic functional groups.

HETEROCYCLIC MOLECULES

Students should be able to:

16. Assign pH characteristics to the common heterocycles and identify the atom(s) responsible for the heterocycles' acidity or basicity.
17. Predict whether the heterocycle is aromatic or not.
18. Predict and draw/identify the structure of instability products (in vitro) of common to heterocycles where appropriate.
19. Predict and draw/identify the structure of metabolic products (in vivo) formed from common heterocycles.

COMPLEX ORGANIC MOLECULES

Students should be able to apply their knowledge of individual organic functional groups and heterocycles to:

20. Predict physical-chemical properties of polyfunctional organic molecules. The physical-chemical properties include water solubility at pH 7 and acidic and basic media, pH characteristics, stereochemical properties, and chemical stability/instability.
21. Predict and draw/identify the structure of metabolic products formed in vivo in polyfunctional organic molecules.

OLIGONUCLEOTIDES AND NUCLEIC ACIDS

Students should be able to:

22. Identify the five bases, the two sugars, and the sites of phosphorylation common to nucleic acids.
23. Discuss the common nomenclature associated with nucleic acids and oligonucleotides.
24. Describe the common physical-chemical properties of nucleic acids and oligonucleotides.
25. Describe the general types of metabolic reactions common to oligonucleotides.

PROTEINS

Students should be able to:

26. Identify the natural occurring amino acids and assign the common abbreviations to each of these amino acids.

27. Discuss the common chemical instabilities (in vitro) of proteins and identify protein-derived instability products.
28. Distinguish between primary, secondary, and tertiary structures of proteins.
29. Predict the common metabolic products (in vivo) formed in proteins and identify the products of metabolism.

Glossary

acid. a substance that can give up or donate a proton (Brønsted-Lowry) or has the ability to accept a pair of electrons (Lewis).

aromatic ring. an exceptionally stable ring system that results from overlapping π electrons, most commonly six π electrons within a five- or six-membered ring.

base. a substance that can donate a pair of electrons (Lewis) or can accept a proton (Brønsted-Lowry).

carbonyl. a carbon doubly-bonded to an oxygen. A carbonyl is not considered an organic functional group, but is part of the following functional groups: ketone, aldehyde, and carboxylic acid and its derivatives.

chiral or chirality. refers to an asymmetric center (usually a carbon with four different substituents) within a structure resulting in two nonsuperimposable structures. These structures are enantiomers of each other.

conjugation reaction. a form of metabolism, normally referred to as a phase 2 metabolism, consisting of glucuronidation, sulfation, acetylation, or methylation.

dipole. unequal sharing of a pair of electrons resulting in a partial negative (δ^-) and partial positive (δ^+) charge within a molecule.

E and Z nomenclature. a nomenclature assigned to isomeric compounds resulting from a lack of free rotation around a double bond or a cyclic ring. When the two top-priority substituents appear on the opposite sides of the molecule the E configuration is assigned (previously *trans* or *anti*), while if the two top-priority groups appear on the same side of the molecule the Z configuration is assigned (previously *cis* or *syn*).

electrophile. electron loving and as such is commonly a positively charged species which will react with an electron-rich substance (nucleophile).

enantiomer. two compounds with the same molecular formula, but which are nonsuperimposable mirror images of each other. They are able to bend plane polarized light to the same degree in opposite directions.

hydrophilic. water loving. Hydrophilic refers to the ability of an organic functional group to bond to water due to the affinity it has for water.

International Union of Pure and Applied Chemistry (IUPAC). the organization responsible for defining and setting the official nomenclature for chemical substances.

intermolecular bonding. chemical bonding between two separate identical or nonidentical molecules.

intramolecular bonding. chemical bonding within a specific molecule.

ion. a formally charged atom that can be either a cation ($+$) or an anion ($-$).

isoforms, protein. different forms of the same protein that can result from various modifications prior to or after formation of the protein.

lipophilic. fat-loving. Lipophilic refers to the affinity that an organic functional group has for an oily or lipid layer such as octanol or a lipid membrane.

nucleophile. nucleus loving and as such is commonly an electron-rich species that reacts with an electron-deficient substance (electrophile).

π Value (for water solubility). hydrophilic-lipophilic value for each functional group. Negative values indicate hydrophilicity and positive values indicate lipophilicity.

"R" and "S" nomenclature. a nomenclature developed by Cahn-Ingold-Prelog to indicate the absolute configuration of an asymmetric center. R (rectus) indicates a clockwise direction in going from the top-priority substituent to the lowest priority substituent, while S (sinister) indicates a counterclockwise direction in going from the top-priority substituent to the lowest priority substituent.

stereoselective. a chemical reaction leading to formation of an asymmetric center in which one isomer is formed preferentially over the second isomer.

solubilizing potential. the extent to which hydrophilic organic functional groups can dissolve a molecule in water. It is normally estimated as the number of carbon atoms that the group can dissolve.

van der Waal forces. also known as dispersion forces or induced dipole-induced dipole attraction. It is an attraction between two molecules resulting from a mutual distortion of electron clouds making up a covalent bond.

xenobiotic. any substance foreign to the human body (most drugs).

Index

Page numbers in italics indicate figures; those followed by t indicate tables.

A

Acetal, 45, *45*
Acetaldehyde, *43*
Acetic acid, *62*
Acetone, *43*
Acetylation, 103, 181t, 182–183
Acetylcholinesterase (AChE) inhibitor, case study, 83–84
Acid
  defined, 30
  reaction of, with base in water, 171–172, 173t
Acid-base chart, 170t
Acid-base pair, conjugate, 167–168, *168*
Acidic organic functional groups, 173–174, 174t
Acidity, 167–175
  of carboxylic acid, 65
  defined, 167–168
  of phenols, 30–32, *31*
  of piperidine, 113
  relative strengths of, 169
  of sulfonamides, 86, *87*
  in water solubility, 161–162, *162*
Acridine, 129, *130*
Adenine, 122–124, *123, 124*
Aerosol dusting products, case study, 21
Alcohol dehydrogenase (ADH), 25, 179
Alcohols
  aldehydes and, chemical reaction between, 44–45
  case studies, 27–28
  ketones and, chemical reaction between, 44–45
  metabolism of, 25–26, *26*
  nomenclature of, 23, *23*
  physical-chemical properties of, 24–25
    boiling points, 24, 24t
    oxidation, 25
    solubility of, 24–25, 24t, 26, 153, 158t
    stability, 25
Aldehyde dehydrogenases, 180
Aldehydes, 42–48
  case studies, 47–48
  hydrazine and, 92, *93*
  metabolic oxidation/reduction reactions of, 178t
  metabolism of, 45–47, *46–47*

  nomenclature of, 42, *43*
  oximes and, 92, *92*
  physical-chemical properties of, 42, 43–45
    boiling points of, 43, 44t
    chemical reactivity of, 44–45
    oxidation of, 44, *44, 46*
    solubility of, 44t, 158t
Alkanes, 6–10
  metabolic oxidation/reduction reactions of, 178t
  metabolism of, 9–10, *10*
  nomenclature of, 6, 6–7
  physical-chemical properties of, 7–9
    boiling points, 7t
    chemical stability, 9
    solubility, 8, *8*
Alkene isomers, 13–15
Alkenes, 11–15
  cycloalkanes, 13–15
  metabolic oxidation/reduction reactions of, 178t
  metabolism of, 13
  nomenclature of, *11,* 11–12
  physical-chemical properties of, 13, *13*
    boiling points, 13
    oxidation, 13, *13*
    solubility, 13
Amides
  metabolic oxidation/reduction reactions of, 178t
  metabolism of, 77–79
  nomenclature of, 76, *76*
  physical-chemical properties of, 77–79
    boiling points of, 77, 77t
    solubility of, 77, 77t, 158t
    stability of, 78
Amidines, 81–82
  physical-chemical properties of, 81–82
Amines, 49–61
  alkyl, 52
  aromatic, 52–53
  case studies, 59–61
  metabolic oxidation/reduction reactions of, 178t
  metabolism of, 55–58
  nomenclature of, 49, 49–50

Amines (Cont.)
  physical-chemical properties of, 50–55
    boiling points of, 50, 51t
    conjugation reactions of, 57, *57*
    dealkylation of, 55–56
    salts of, 53–55, *55*
    solubility of, 50, 51t, 158t, 159, *159*
    quaternary ammonium salts, 58–59
Amino acids (*See also* Proteins)
  conformational changes, 146, 147–148,
    147–148
  deamidation reactions of, *145,* 145–146
  hydrogen bonding of, 147–148, *147–148*
  hydrolysis reaction of, 146, *146*
  oxidation reactions of, 144, *144–145*
  in proteins, 141
  racemization reaction of, 146, *147*
  structures of various, 143t
4-Aminobenzene sulfonamide, *87*
Aminoglycoside, antibiotics, 45
2-Aminopropane, *49*
Ampicillin, case study, 60–61
Amyl nitrite, 91, *91*
Angiotensin-converting enzyme (ACE) inhibitor,
  case study, 71–72
Anisole, *36, 38*
Anthracene, *16*
Anthracycline anticancer drugs, case study, 59–60
Antihistamines, case study, 70
Antisense drugs, 133, 134, 136
ARA C, *115*
Arachidonic acid, 64
Arginine, 81
Arginine vasopressin (AVP), *142,* 149, *150*
Aromatic hydrocarbons, 16–18
  metabolism of, 17–18, *18*
  nomenclature of, 16, *16*
  physical-chemical properties of, 16–17
    hydroxylation, 16
Arylamine, 90
Aryl nitro groups
  metabolism of, 90, *91*
Aryl sulfonamides
  nomenclature of, 86, *87*
  physical-chemical properties of, 86
Aspartate (Asp), 146, *146, 147*
Asymmetric molecules, 164–166
Atorvastatin, *103*
ATP, *124*
Aziridine, 98–99, *99*
AZT, 101

B

Barbiturates, 117, 118, *118*
Barbituric acid, 117–119, *118*
Base

defined, 50
  reaction of acid with, in water, 171–172,
    173t
  strength of, 50–51
  strong, 51
  weak, 51
Basicity, 167–175
  of amidines, 81–82, *82*
  of amines, 50–53, *51, 52*
  of carboxylic acids, 67–68
  defined, 167–168
  electrons and, *51, 52*
  of guanidines, 81–82, *82*
  of pyridine, 113
  relative strengths of, 169–170
  in water solubility, 161, *162*
Basic organic functional groups, 174–175, 175t
Benzene, *16*
Benzene sulfonamide, *87*
Benzene sulfonic acid, *85*
Benzimidazole, 122, *122*
Benzodiazepines, *128,* 128–129
Benzopyrroles, 120–121, *121*
Benzothiadiazine-1,1-dioxide, *127,* 127–128, *128*
Benzothiazole, *122*
Benzoxazole, *122*
Benzylpenicillin, case study, 60–61
Beta-lactam, 76, *76,* 99–100, *100*
  hydrolysis of, 100, *100*
Bicyclic heterocycles
  five-membered ring plus six-membered
    four heteroatoms, 122–124, *123, 124*
    nitrogen, 120–121, *121*
    ring, 120–124
    two heteroatoms, 121–122, *122*
  six-membered ring plus seven-membered
    ring, *128,* 128–129
  six-membered ring plus six-membered ring
    nitrogen, 125, *125,* 127, *127*
    oxygen, 125–126, *126*
    sulfur, 126–128, *127, 128*
Boiling points
  of alcohols, 24, 24t
  of aldehyde, 43, 44t
  of alkanes, 7t
  of alkenes, 13
  of amides, 77, 77t
  of amines, 50, 51t
  of carboxylic acids, 65
  of esters, 74, 74t
  of ethers, 36–37, *37*
  of halogenated hydrocarbon, 20
  of ketones, 43, 44t
  of *n*-hexane, 7t
  of phenols, 30, 30t, 31
  of thioethers, 38

of various carboxylic acids, 63t
Bonding, 1–5
    cation-π, 5, 5
    covalent, 2, 2
    dipole-dipole, 2–3, 3
    hydrogen, 2–3, 3
    ion-dipole, 4, 4–5
    ionic attraction, 3, 3–4
2-Bromo-4-methylpentane, 19, 19
Buprenorphine, case study, 162–163
iso-Butane, 6
N-Butane, 6, 7t
2-Butanone, 43
cis-2-Butene, 12
trans-2-Butene, 12
t-Butyl acetate, 73
tert-Butyl alcohol, 23
Butylbarbital, metabolism of, 10
1-Butylene, 11
iso-Butylene, 11
t-Butylethylmethylamine, 49
N-Butyliodide, 19
t-Butyl phenyl carbonate, 79
Butyric acid
    ethanol and, chemical bonding between, 66

C

Caproic acid, 62
Carbamates, 79–81, 158t, 178t
    metabolism of, 80–81, 81
    nomenclature of, 79, 80
    physical-chemical properties of, 80
Carbolic acid, 29
Carbonates, 79–81, 158t, 178t
    metabolism of, 80–81, 81
    nomenclature of, 79, 79
    physical-chemical properties of, 80
Carbontetrachloride, 19
    flammability of, 20
Carbonyl, defined, 42
Carboxylic acids, 43
    carbonyl, 65
    case studies, 70–72
    conjugation reactions of, 68–69, 69
    functional derivatives of, 73–84
        amides, 76–79
        amidines and guanidines, 81–82
        carbonates, carbamates, and ureas,
            79–81
        case studies, 82–84
        esters, 73–75
    metabolism of, 68–69
    nomenclature of, 62, 62–65
    physical-chemical properties of, 65–68
        acidity of, 65
        basicity of, 67–68

boiling points of, 63t, 65
    solubility of, 65, 158t
Catechol, 29
Cation-π, bonding, 5, 5
Cefdinir, 92
Cefixime, case study, 94–95
Ceftizoxime, 109
Celecoxib, 108
Cephalosporin, 99, 100
Chemical reactivity
    of aldehydes, 44–45
    of ketones, 44–45
    of phenols, 32, 32
Chemical stability, of alkanes, 9
Chiral center, 165
Chirality, 165
Chiral molecules, 9
Chloramphenicol, case study, 94–95
Chlordiazepoxide, 128
Chloroform, 19, 20
    oxidation of, 20, 20
Chloroquine, 125
Chlorothiazide, 127
Chlorpromazine, 38, 39, 130
Chlorpropamide, 87
Chlorzoxazone, 122
Cimetidine, 38
Ciprofloxacin, 119
Clonidine, 81
Coenzyme A (CoA), 69
Combivir, case study, 139–140
Conformational isomers, 14–15, 15
Congestive heart failure (CHF), 59
Conjugate acid-base pair, 167–168, 168
Conjugated estrogens, case study, 35
Conjugation reactions, 180–183, 181t
    acetylation, 181t, 182–183
    of amines, 57, 57
    of carboxylic acids, 68–69, 69
    glucuronidation, 180–182, 181t
    methylation, 181t, 183
    sulfation, 181t, 182
Corticosteroid ointment, case study, 48
Coumarin, 125–126, 126
o-Cresol, 29
Cycloalkanes, 13–15
Cyclohexane, 14, 14
Cyclohexanol, 30
Cyclopentane, 14, 14
Cyclopropane, 13, 14
CYP450 catalyzed reactions, 177–178, 178t
Cysteines, 144, 144, 148
Cytidine-5'-monophosphate (CMP), 116
Cytidylic acid, 116
Cytochrome P450, 17, 176–178
Cytosine, 114–117, 115

D

Dealkylation
  of amines, 55–56, 177
  of ethers, 38, *38*, 177
  metabolic, 38, *38*, 39, *39*
  of piperidine, 113
  of thioethers, 39, *39*
Deamidation reactions, of amino acids, *145*,
  145–146
Demethylation, of amines, 55
Deoxyadenylate, *124*
Deoxyribonucleic acid (DNA) (*See* Nucleic acids
  deoxyribonucleic acid (DNA))
Deoxyuridylic acid, 116, *116*
Desimipramine, 55
Diamine oxidase (DAO), 56
Diazepam, 128
Diazines, 114, *114*
Dibenzazepine, 127
Diethylether, *36*
1,2-Dihydroxybenzene, 29
1,3-Dihydroxybenzene, 29
1,4-Dihydroxybenzene, 29
3,3-Dimethylbutanal, *43*
Dimethylketone, *43*
2,4-Dimethyl-4-phenylpentanoic acid, 62
Diphenhydramine, glucuronidation of, 58
Dipole-dipole bonding, 2–3, *3*
Dipole-induced dipole attraction, 2
5,5-disubstituted barbituric acids, 118, *118*, *119*
DNA polymerase, case study, 138–139
Docosahexaenoic acid (DHA), 64
Drug-drug interactions, 177–178, 178t
Drug interactions, cytochrome P450 and,
  177–178, 178t
Drug metabolism, 176–183
  conjugation reactions (*See* Conjugation
    reactions)
  defined, 176
  hydrolase enzymes, 180
  oxygenase enzymes (*See* Oxygenase
    enzymes)
Drugs
  phenolate salts and, 32
  solubility of, 1

E

Eicosapentaenoic acid (EPA), 64
Electrons, basicity and, *51*, 52
Emulsions, case study, 163
Enantiomeric forms, of molecules, 9
Enantiomers, 164–165, *165*
Enzymes
  metabolic (*See* Metabolic enzymes)
  protein hydrolyzing, 149, 150t

Epothilone B, case study, 82–83
Epoxides, 17, 96–98, *98*
Essential fatty acids, 64
Esterase, 80
Esters, 73–76
  metabolic oxidation/reduction reactions of,
    178t
  metabolism of, 75, *75*
  nomenclature of, 73, *73*
  physical-chemical properties of, 73–75
    boiling points of, 74, 74t
    solubility of, 74, 74t, 158t
Ethanal, *43*
Ethane, *6*
Ethanoic acid, *62*
Ethanol, 23, 65–66
  butyric acid and, chemical bonding between,
    66
Ether anesthetics, case study, 41
Ethers
  case studies, 40–41
  metabolic oxidation/reduction reactions of,
    178t
  metabolism of, 38, *38*
  nomenclature of, 36, *36*
  physical-chemical properties of, 36–37, *37*
    boiling points, 36–37, *37*
    oxidation, 37
    solubility of, 36–37, *37*, 158t, 159, *159*
Ethoxyethane, *36*
Ethoxzolamide, *122*
Ethyl alcohol, 23
Ethylchloride, *19*
4-Ethyl-2,7-dimethyloctane, 6–7, *7*
Ethylene, *11*
Ethylene chloride, *19*
Ethyl isopropyl carbonate, 79
Ethylmethylamine, *49*
Ethylmethylether, *36*
Ethylmethylketone, *43*
N-Ethyl-N-methyl-2-methyl-2-aminopropane,
  49
Ethyl 2-propyl carbonate, 79

F

Five-membered ring heterocycles
  complex, 109–112
  nitrogen, 102–103, *103*
  oxygen, 100–102, *101*, *102*
  sulfur, *104*, 104–105, *105*
  with two or more heteroatoms, 105–112
Flavin monooxygenase (FMO), 39, 56, 179
Fluconazole, *111*
5-Fluorouridine-2'-deoxyribosyl phosphate
  (5-FUDR), 117, *117*

5-Fluorouridine monophosphate (5-FUMP), 117, *117*
FMO (*See* Flavin monooxygenase (FMO))
Formaldehyde, *43*
Formamide, 77
Formic acid, *62*
Four-membered ring heterocycle, 99–100, *100*
5-FU, *115*, 117
Furans, 100–101, *101*
Furosemide (Lasix), *101*
    case study, 130–131

G

Glucuronic acid, 45, *46*
Glucuronidation, 180–182, 181t
    of diphenhydramine, *58*
Guanidines, 81–82
    physical-chemical properties of, 81–82
Guanine, 122–123, *123*

H

Halogenated hydrocarbons, 19–22
    case studies, 21–22
    metabolism of, *20*, 20–21
    nomenclature of, 19, *19*
    physical-chemical properties of, 19–20, *20*
        boiling points, 20
        flammability, 20
        oxidation, 20, *20*
        solubility, 20
H_2 antagonists, case study, 93–94
Hemiacetal, formation and instability, 45
Hemiketal, formation and instability, 45
N-Heptane, 7t
Heteroatom
    defined, 96
    prefixes for, 97t
Heterocycles, 96–132
    bicyclic (*See* Bicyclic heterocycles)
    case studies, 130–132
    defined, 96
    five-membered ring
        complex, 109–112
        nitrogen, 102–103, *103*
        oxygen, 100–102, *101, 102*
        sulfur, *104*, 104–105, *105*
        with two or more heteroatoms, 105–112
    four-membered ring, 99–100, *100*
    seven- and eight-membered ring, 120, *120*
    six-membered ring, 112–113, *113*
        saturated, 119, *119*
        suffixes for, 97t
        with two heteroatoms, 114–119
    three-membered ring, 96–99
        nitrogen, 98–99, *99*

oxygen, 96–98, 97t, *98*
    tricyclic, 129–130, *130*
Hexahydroazepine, 120, *120*
N-Hexane
    boiling point of, 7t
    solubility of, *8*
Hexanoic acid, *62*
Histidine, 144, *145*
Hydantoin nucleus, 110
Hydantoins, *111*, 112, *112*
Hydralazine, *93*
Hydrazide, 92, *93*
Hydrazine, 92, *93*
    and aldehyde, 92, *93*
    and ketone, 92, *93*
Hydrazone, 92, *93*
Hydrocarbons
    aromatic (*See* Aromatic hydrocarbons)
    halogenated (*See* Halogenated
        hydrocarbons)
Hydrochloric acid, 54
Hydrochlorothiazide, 87
Hydrogen bonding, 2–3, *3*
    of amino acids, 147–148, *147–148*
    of carboxylic acids, 65
    between ethanol and water, 24, *24*
    intramolecular, 161, *161*
Hydrolase enzymes, 180
Hydrolysis
    of beta-lactam, 100, *100*
    of organic nitrates, 91, *91*
    of peptides, 149, 150t
Hydrolysis reaction, of amino acids, 146, *146*
Hydrophilic-lipophilic values, 160, 160t
Hydrophilic molecule, defined, 1
Hydrophobic molecule, defined, 1
Hydroquinone, 29
Hydroxylamine, 90, 92, *92*
Hydroxylation
    aromatic, 16–17, *17*, 124, *124*

I

Imidazole, 107–109, *108*
Imidazolidine, 107, *108, 109*
Imidazoline, 107, 109
2-Imidazoline, 107, *108*
Imine, 92
Imipramine, 55, *130*
Indole, 120–121, *121*
Induced dipole attraction, 2
Intermolecular bonding (*See* Bonding)
International Union of Pure and Applied
        Chemistry (IUPAC) (*See also* specific
        organic group)

International Union of Pure and Applied
Chemistry (IUPAC) (Cont.)
nomenclature of, 6, 6–7
Intramolecular hydrogen bonding (IMHB),
161, 161
Ion-dipole bonding, 4, 4–5
Ionic attraction, 3, 3–4
Isoindole, 120–121, 121
Isomers, 12, 164–165
alkene, 13–15
cis, 12, 15
conformational, 14–15, 15
diazine, 114, 114
geometric, 12
trans, 12, 15
Isoniazid, 93
Isopropyl alcohol, 23
Isopropylamine, 49
Isopropyl propionate, 73
Isoquinoline, 125, 125
Isosorbide dinitrate, 91
Isoxazole, 105, 105–106, 107
IUPAC (International Union of Pure and
Applied Chemistry) (See also specific
organic group)
nomenclature of, 6, 6–7
Ixabepilone (Ixempra), case study, 82–83

K
Ketones, 42–48
case studies, 47–48
hydrazine and, 92, 93
metabolism of, 45–47, 46–47
nomenclature of, 42, 43
oximes and, 92, 92
physical-chemical properties of, 42, 43–45
boiling points of, 43, 44t
chemical reactivity of, 44–45
oxidation of, 44, 44, 46
solubility of, 44t, 158t

L
Lactam, 76, 76
Lactone, 73, 74, 125–126
Lamivudine (3TC), case study, 139–140
Levorphanol, case study, 162–163
Linezolid, 111
Linoleic acid, 64
Linolenic acid, 64
Lipophilic molecule, defined, 1
Lipophobic molecule, defined, 1
Log P, 160–162
Losartan, 111
LSD, 121
Lunamine, case study, 21

M
Mechlorethamine, 99, 99
Meperidine, 113
Meprobamate, metabolism of, 10
Meropenem, 100
Messenger RNA (mRNA), 133, 136, 141 (See
also Nucleic acids)
Mesylates, 85, 85
Metabolic dealkylation, 38, 38, 39, 39
Metabolic enzymes, 176–183
conjugation reactions, 180–183, 181t
acetylation, 181t, 182–183
glucuronidation, 180–182, 181t
methylation, 181t, 183
sulfation, 181t, 182
hydrolase enzymes, 180
oxygenase enzymes, 176–180
alcohol dehydrogenase, 179
aldehyde dehydrogenase, 180
cytochrome P450, 176–178
flavin monooxygenase, 179
Metabolic oxidation, 39, 39
Metabolism
of alcohol, 25–26, 26
phases, 25–26, 26
of aldehydes, 45–47, 46–47
of alkanes, 9–10, 10
of alkenes, 13
of amides, 77–79
of amines, 55–58
of aromatic hydrocarbons, 17–18, 18
of aryl nitro groups, 90, 91
of butylbarbital, 10
of carbamates, 80–81, 81
of carbonates, 80–81, 81
of carboxylic acids, 68–69, 70
of esters, 75, 75
of ethers, 38, 38
of halogenated hydrocarbons, 20, 20–21
of ketones, 45–47, 46–47
of meprobamate, 10
of nucleic acids, 136, 137
of oligonucleotides, 136, 137
of phenols, 33, 33
of proteins, 148–150
of pyrimidine, 116, 116–117, 117
of thioethers, 39, 39
of ureas, 80–81
xenobiotic, 176
Methadone maintenance program, case study,
47
Methanal, 43
Methane, 6
Methane sulfonic acid, 85, 85
Methanoic acid, 62

Methanol, 23
Methapyrilene, 104
Methionine, 144
Methoxybenzene, 36
2-Methoxy-4,4-dimethylpentane, 36
Methoxyethane, 36
Methyl alcohol, 23
N-Methylaminoethane, 49
Methylation, 33, 181t, 183
Methylation reaction, 57, 57
4-Methylbenzene sulfonamide, 87
Methylene chloride, 19
Methylfluoride, 19
N-Methyl-N-isopropylvaleramide, 76
N-Methyl-N-phenylbenzamide, 76
N-Methyl-N-2-propylpentanamide, 76
2-Methylphenol, 29
Methylphenylether, 36
Methylphenylketone, 43
2-Methyl-2-propanol, 23
2-Methyl-2-propyl ethanoate, 73
6-Methylthiopurine, 38, 39
5-methyluracil, 114–117, 115
Metronidazole, 90, 108
Mevalonic acid, 62, 63
Monoamine oxidase (MAO), 56
Monomethoxy polyethylene glycol, case study, 152
Monounsaturated fatty acids, 63–64
Morphine, case study, 162–163
Morpholine, 119, 119

N
Naphthalene, 16
Nicotine, 103
Nitrate group, 90–91, 91
Nitrazapam, 90
Nitrite group, 91, 91
Nitrogen
    in five-membered ring heterocycles, 102–103, 103
    in five-membered ring heterocycles with two or more heteroatoms, 105–109, 105–109
    in five-membered ring plus six-membered bicyclic heterocycles, 120–121, 121
    functional groups
        case studies, 93–95
        hydrazide, 92, 93
        hydrazine, 92, 93
        hydrazone, 92, 93
        nitrate, 90–91, 91
        nitrite, 91, 91
        nitro, 90
        oximes, 92, 92
    oxidation of tertiary amine, 56, 56

    in six-membered ring heterocycles, 112–113, 113
    in six-membered ring plus seven-membered ring bicyclic heterocycle, 128, 128–129
    in six-membered ring plus six-membered ring bicyclic heterocycles, 125, 125, 127, 127
    in three-membered ring heterocycles, 98–99, 99
Nitrogen mustards, 98
Nitroglycerin, 90–91, 91
Nitro group, 90, 90
4-Nitrophenol, 29
p-Nitrophenol, 29
Norepinephrine bitartrate, case study, 34
Nucleic acids, 133–140
    case studies, 138–140
    metabolism of, 136, 137
    nomenclature of, 133–134
    physical-chemical properties of, 135, 135–136, 136, 137
    structure of, 135
Nucleic acids deoxyribonucleic acid (DNA) (See also Nucleic acids)
    functions of, 133
    nomenclature of, 133–134
    physical-chemical properties of, 135–136
Nucleoside, 133, 134
Nucleotides, 133, 134

O
Octahydroazocine, 120, 120
N-Octane, 7t
Oleaginous ointment (See Corticosteroid ointment, case study)
Oleic acid, 64
Oligonucleotides, 133–140
    case studies, 138–140
    functions of, 133–134
    metabolism of, 136, 137
    physical-chemical properties of, 135, 135–136, 136, 137
    ribose, 136, 137
Omega fatty acids, 64
Omeprazole, 122
Opioids, case study, 40, 162–163
Organic nitrates, 90, 91
Oxazole, 105, 105–106, 107
Oxazolidinones, 110–111, 111, 112
Oxidation
    of alcohols, 25, 25
    of aldehydes, 44, 44, 46
    of alkenes, 13, 13
    of carboxylic acids, 69, 69
    of chloroform, 20, 20

Oxidation (Cont.)
  of ethers, 37
  of ketones, 44, 44
  metabolic, 39, 39
  nitrogen, of tertiary amine, 56, 56
  of phenols, 32, 33
  of thioethers, 39, 39
  of thiol group, 39–40
Oxidation reactions, of amino acids, 144,
    144–145
Oxidation reductions, in protein metabolism,
    148, 149
Oximes, 92, 92
  and aldehydes, 92, 92
  and ketones, 92, 92
Oxiranes, 96–98, 97t, 98
Oxolane, 101
Oxole, 101
Oxygen
  in five-membered ring heterocycles,
    100–102, 101, 102
  in five-membered ring heterocycles with two
    or more heteroatoms, 105–107, 105–107
  in six-membered ring plus six-membered
    ring bicyclic heterocycles, 125–126, 126
  in three-membered ring heterocycles, 96–98,
    97t, 98
Oxygenase enzymes, 176–180
  alcohol dehydrogenase, 179
  aldehyde dehydrogenase, 180
  cytochrome P450, 176–178
  flavin monooxygenase, 179
Oxytocin, case study, 151

P

Palmitoleic acid, 64
Paradimethylaminobenzaldehyde, 158, 158
Pegasys, case study, 152
Peg-interferon alfa-2a, case study, 152
Penicillin, 100
Pentaerythritol tetranitrate, case study, 94–95
N-Pentane, 7t
Pentazocine, 120
Peptides, hydrolysis of, 149, 150t
Peroxides, 37, 37
Phenanthrene, 16
Phenmetrazine, 119
Phenobarbital, 118
Phenols
  case studies, 34–35
  metabolism of, 33, 33
  nomenclature of, 29, 29
  physical-chemical properties of, 29–32, 30t,
    31–33
    acidity, 30–32, 31

boiling points, 30, 30t, 31
    chemical reactivity, 32, 32
    oxidation, 32, 33
    salt formation, 32
    solubility of, 30, 30t, 31, 158t, 159, 159
Phenothiazine, 129, 130
Phentolamine, 81
Phenylethanolamine-N-methyltransferase
    (PNMT), 57
1-Phenylethanone, 43
Phenylethylamine, case study, 27
Phenyl 2-methyl-2-propyl carbonate, 79
N-Phenyl-N-(2-propyl)-2-aminopentane, 49
Phenytoin, 111
Phosgene, 20
Piperazine, 119, 119
Piperidine, 112–113, 113
Polythiazide, 127
Polyunsaturated fatty acids, 64
Praziquantel, 125
Prazosin, 127
Premarin, case study, 35
Procaine, 161–162, 162
Propanal, 43
Propane, 6, 7t
Propanoic acid, 62
2-Propanol, 23
2-Propanone, 43
Propionaldehyde, 43
Propionic acid, 62
Propylbromide, 19
Propylene, 11
2-Propyl propanoate, 73
Protein hydrolyzing enzymes, 149, 150t
Proteins, 141–152 (See also Amino acids)
    case studies, 151–152
    metabolism of, 148–150
      hydrolysis of peptides, 149, 150t
      oxidation reductions, 148, 149
    nomenclature of, 141, 142
    physical-chemical properties of, 141–148
      conformational changes, 146, 147–148,
        147–148
      deamidation reactions, 145, 145–146
      hydrolysis reaction, 146, 146
      oxidation reactions, 144, 144–145
      racemization reaction, 146, 147
Psychastigmine, case study, 83–84
Pteridine, 126, 127
Purine, 122–124, 123, 124
Pyrazine, 114
Pyrazole, 107–109, 108
Pyridazine, 114
Pyridine, 112–114, 113
Pyrimethamine, case study, 88–89

Pyrimidine, *114,* 114–119
  metabolism of, *116,* 116–117, *117*
  nomenclature of, 114, *115,* 117, *118*
  physical-chemical properties of, 114–116,
    115, 117–119, *118–119*

Q

Quaternary ammonium salts, 58–59
  nomenclature of, 58
  physical-chemical properties of, 58–59
Quinazoline, 126, *127*
Quinocrine, *130*
Quinoline, 125, *125*

R

Racemization reaction, of amino acids, 146, *147*
Resorcinol, *29*
Ribonucleic acid (RNA) (*See also* Nucleic acids)
  functions of, 133
  nomenclature of, 133–134
  physical-chemical properties of, 136
  uracil in synthesis of, *116,* 116–117
Ribose oligonucleotides, 136, *137*
Rifampin, *93*
Rivastigmine, case study, 83–84
Rosiglitazone, *113*

S

S-adenosylmethionine (SAM), 33, 57
Salts
  of amines, 53–55, *55*
  of carboxylic acids, 68
  of 5,5-disubstituted barbituric acids, *119*
  of phenols, 32
  quaternary ammonium, 58–59
  of sulfonamide, 86, *87*
SAM (*See* S-adenosylmethionine (SAM))
Schiff base, 92
Six-membered ring heterocycles, 112–113, *113*
  saturated, 119, *119*
  with two heteroatoms, 114–119
Sodium chloride, solubility of, 8, *8*
Solubility, 1–5, 153–163, 158t
  of alcohol, 24–25, 24t, 26, 153, 158t
  of aldehydes, 44t, 158t
  of alkenes, 13
  of amides, 77, 77t, 158t
  of amines, 50, 51t, 158t, 159, *159*
  of carboxylic acids, 65, 158t
  dipole-dipole bonding, 2–3, *3*
  of drugs, 1
  of esters, 74, 74t, 158t
  of ethers, 36–37, *37,* 158t, 159, *159*
  of halogenated hydrocarbon, 20
  ion-dipole bonding, *4,* 4–5

  ionic attraction, *3,* 3–4
  of ketones, 44t, 158t
  key to, 1
  of *n*-hexane, *8*
  of phenols, 30, 30t, 31, 158t, 159, *159*
  predicting, 153–163
    analytic method for, 160–162
    case studies, 162–163
    chemical bonding, 153–156
    empiric method for, 156–159
  of sodium chloride, 8, *8*
  of sulfonic acids, 86t
  of thioethers, 39
  van der Waals forces, 2, *2*
  of various carboxylic acids, 63t
Stability
  of alcohol, 25
  of amides, 78
  of carboxylic acids, 66
Stereoisomerism, 9, *9,* 164–166
Substituted barbiturates, 117, *118, 119*
Sufentanil, *104*
Sulfadiazine, case study, 88–89
Sulfamethizole, *110*
Sulfation, 181t, 182
Sulfisoxazole, *87*
Sulfonamides
  acidity of, 86, *87*
  case study, 87–88
  nomenclature of, 86, *87*
  physical-chemical properties of, 86
Sulfone, 178t
Sulfonic acids
  nomenclature of, 85, *85*
  physical-chemical properties of, 85
  solubility of, 86t
Sulfoxide, 178t
Sulfur
  in five-membered ring heterocycles, *104,*
    104–105, *105*
  in five-membered ring heterocycles with two
    or more heteroatoms, 109, *109*
  in six-membered ring plus six-membered
    ring bicyclic heterocycles, 126–128,
    127, 128
Symmetric molecules, 164, *164*

T

Taxane therapy, case study, 27
Tetraethyl ammonium (TEA) sulfate, 58
Tetrahydrofuran, 100–102, *101, 102*
Tetrahydrothiophene, 104, *104, 105*
2,5,7,7-Tetramethyl-4-octanone, *43*
Tetrazoles, 110, *111*
Thiadiazole, 110, *110*

Thiazide diuretics, *127*, 127–128, *128*
1,3-Thiazole, 109, *109*
Thiazolsulfone, *109*
Thienamycin, *100*
Thioethers, 178t
    metabolism of, 39, *39*
    nomenclature of, 38, *38*
    physical-chemical properties of, 38–39
Thiol, 178t
Thiol oxidation, 39–40
Thiophene, 104, *104*
Three-membered ring heterocycles
    nitrogen, 98–99, *99*
    oxygen, 96–98, 97t, *98*
Thymidylic acid, 116, *116*
Thymine, 114–116, *115*
Timolol, *110*
Tolazamide, *120*
p-Toluene sulfonamide, *87*
p-Toluene sulfonic acid, *85*
Triamterene, *127*
Triazoles, 110, *111*
Tricyclic heterocycles, 129–130, *130*
Trifluorothymidine, *115*
3,6,6-Trimethyl-3-heptene, *11*, 11–12
Tryptophan, 144, *145*
Tyrosine, 144, *145*, 156, *157*

U
UDP-glucuronosyltransferase (UGT)
    in alcohol metabolism, 26
UGT (*See* UDP-glucuronosyltransferase (UGT))
Uracil, 114–116, *115*

Ureas, 79–81, 158t
    metabolism of, 80–81
    nomenclature of, 79, *80*
    physical-chemical properties of, 80
Uric acid, 124, *124*
    case study, 131–132
Uridylic acid, 116, *116*

V
Van der Waals forces, 2, *2*

W
Warfarin, 125–126, *126*
Water
    acid-base properties of, 171
    reaction of acid with base in, 171–172, 173t
Water solubility (*See* Solubility)
Watson-Crick model, 135

X
Xanthine, *123*, 123–124, *124*
Xenobiotic metabolism, 176
Xenobiotics, 176

Z
Zidovudine (ZDV), case study, 139–140
Zwitterion, 157, *157*